Painless Pregnancy

Painless Pregnancy

Parvesh Handa

Exceptional Assistance & Contributions by

Dr D.S. Jaspal
National Vice Chairman, Indian Medical Association

Tips from

Dr Reeta Jaspal
Senior Gynecologist & President IMA - Haryana

Vij Books India Pvt Ltd
New Delhi (India)

Published by

Vij Books India Pvt Ltd
(Publishers, Distributors & Importers)
2/19 (Second Floor), Ansari Road, Darya Ganj
New Delhi - 110002
Phones: 91-11-43596460, 91-11- 65449971
Fax: 91-11-47340674
web: www.vijbooks.com
e-mail : vijbooks@rediffmail.com

ISBN: 978-93-80177-82-3
Price: ₹ 250.00

Printed in India
at Narula Printers , Delhi

CONTENTS

Foreword vii

1 Know Your Body 1

2 Disorders Before Conceiving 12

3 Abnormalities of Genital Organs 26

4 Methods of Family Planning 32

5 Signs and Symptoms of Pregnancy & Abortion 39

6 Types of Pregnancy 45

7 Physical Examination During Pregnancy 55

8 40 Weeks of Pregnancy 62

9 Important Tips During Pregnancy 84

10 Warning Signs During Pregnancy 97

11 Genital Diseases During Pregnancy 103

12 Planning for a Healthy Child? 114

13 Problematic Deliveries 122

14 Venereal Diseases 128

15 Skin Diseases Associated With Pregnancy 136

16 Stages of Labor 143

Important Tips for Mother & Child 160

18 Breasts & Breastfeeding 174

19 Beautiful Body & Pregnancy 185

20 All About Menstruation Menopause & Anemia 210

Disclaimer

This book is not intended to take the place of medical advice from a trained medical professional. Readers are advised to consult a qualified doctor or a gynecologist regarding treatment of their medical problem. Neither the author or publisher takes any responsibility for any possible consequences from any treatment, action or application of medicine,, herb or preparation to any person reading or following the information in this book.

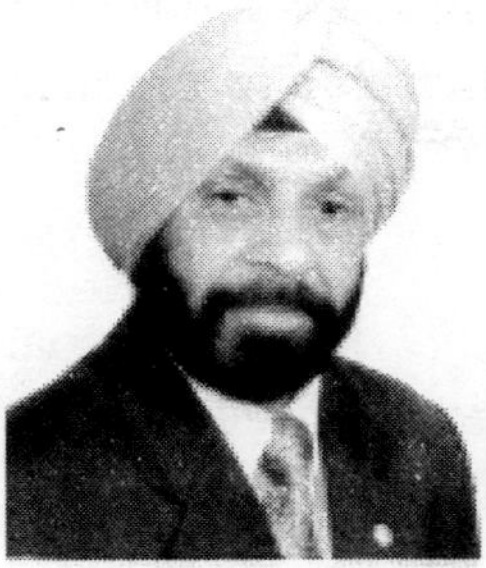

Foreword

The birth of a baby is the birth of a family and a joyous event. This book by Ms Parvesh Handa would educate all those women going to be mother first time and provide a practical guide to painless childbirth. Care has been taken to help expecting mothers and their partners to learn what they need to make good decisions, adopt techniques for a painless pregnancy and pleasant childbearing period. This book would enhance relationship between expecting mother and her companion gain the information, skill, confidence and active participants in their own care.

The psychomotor skills, such as simple exercises and practice of yoga postures, relaxation, labor positions and comfort measures are a vital part of preparation for childbirth. It is hoped, readers would find it enjoyable as they use it to prepare for a safe and joyful birth and confident family beginning. Pregnancy is a state that lasts about nine months when a unborn baby is transforming into a person capable of life outside the safe, protective and totally sufficient environment of the mother's body. The birth process follows three stages of pregnancy, followed by labour and delivery of the child thereby providig complete transition from pregnancy parenthood.

Remember, pregnancy is not a disease, although at this time of extra demand on body, one is more vulnerable to medical complications than at other times in life.

Dr D.S. Jaspal
National Vice President
Indian Medical Association

1

Know Your Body

Every woman on way to become a mother should know about her body thoroughly. There are several women, some of them going to be married or are expectant mothers but they have least knowledge of their own body organs. Most of the teenagers and even newly married women feel hesitant to question about male or female genitals organs, though their knowledge is essential for every one to make married life and pregnancy more enjoyable and healthy, and also allay fears and misconception.

The vulva: The vulva is an ill-defined area, which in gynecological practice comprises the whole of the external genitalia including the perineum. A woman's perineum includes the pelvic floor muscles, external genitalia, urethra, anus and perineal body – the area between the vagina and anus. The external genitalia include the vaginal opening, clitoris, labia majora, labia minora and mono pubis – fatty tissue over the pubic bone. The mons pubis is the only part of the genital organ visible when the woman is in the upright posture, with a cushion of fat in front covered after puberty with more or less short curly hair. The mons pubis is continued in a backward direction into the two outer lips of the vulva (called labia majora). At puberty, hair appears at the outer surface of the labia majora and in some cases on the skin of the perineum as well. The inner surface of the labia majora is soft, moist, pinkish colored and hairless. The skin here contains sebaceous glands, sweat glands and hair follicles. The skin of labia majora is liable to common skin disorders such as lesions, boils and cysts. The labia minora lie on the inner aspect of the labia majora – a thin fold of skin, which do not contain sebaceous glands or hair follicles but have veins and elastic tissue, which erect during sexual activity.

Bartholin's gland is a compound gland measuring about 10 mm. in diameter and about 25 mm. long, which secrete lubricating mucus during coitus. The clitoris consists of a glans covered by the prepuce and a body which is subcutaneous and corresponds to the penis and is attached to the under surface of the pubis. The clitoris is extremely sensitive and during coitus it becomes erect and plays a considerable part in inducing the orgasm of the female. The vaginal orifice is surrounded by hymen. In virgins the hymen is surrounded by thin membrane covering the surface.

The Uterus: The womb is the compartment of female body in which a baby forms and grows till birth. It is also termed as uterus, a pear-shaped hollow thick walled muscular organ situated in the pelvis behind the bladder and in front of the rectum, deep in the lower abdomen. Uterus is divided into two parts – an upper part called the body and the lower part called the cervix, which protrudes into the vagina, the stretchy canal connecting the internal and external genitalia. The uterus is usually of size 3"x2"x1" when in non-pregnant state and it stretches gradually in size to accommodate a fully formed baby. The size and shape of the normal uterus varies throughout the life. An infantile uterus ranges from 2 to 3.3 cm. in length with the cervix accounting for two third of the total length and 0.5 to 1 cm. in diameter. As the puberty approaches, the uterus gradually increases in size with more pronounced growth in the body to the eventual adult pear-shaped appearance. Congenital uterine abnormalities occur in approximately 0.5% of females and associated with increased incidence of abortion and other obstetric complications. Sonogram or an ultrasound may detect anomalies of the uterus. The fallopian tubes extend from the upper sides of the uterus towards the ovaries. Two ovaries located on each side of the uterus are a woman's sex glands, which produce estrogen and progesterone – the female sex hormones. During adolescence, along with hormones from the pituitary and adrenal glands, estrogen stimulates the development of secondary sexual characteristics in the female such as enlarged breasts, body hair. The ovaries also ripen and expel ova (eggs). Out of thousands of ova present in the ovaries, only 400 to 450 are ovulated in a woman's lifetime.

How conception and pregnancy take place?: The question arises, how conception take place and pregnancy develops. After sexual intercourse, sperm travel from vagina through the cervix into the cavity of the uterus and along the fallopian tubes. Conception takes place when a single sperm penetrates or fertilizes an ovum, forming a single cell. At the moment a woman becomes pregnant, a new life begins. Although, large numbers of sperm ejaculate and reach

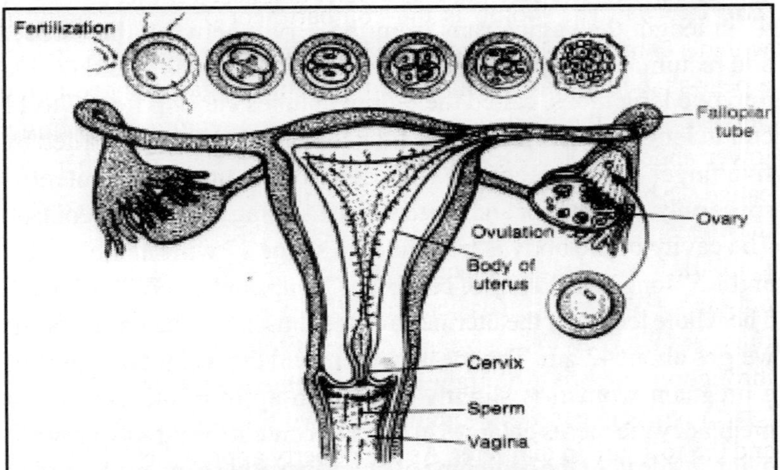

Becoming Pregnant - Conception

the ovum, only one penetrates it. Once ovum is fertilized, a chemical reaction occurs, preventing other sperm from penetrating it. After fertilization, which takes place in the outer one-third of the fallopian tube, the ovum travels along the fallopian tube and embeds within the lining of the uterus. Each ovum and sperm contains 23 chromosomes - the full component of 46 chromosomes, which combine to give the baby unique inherited characteristics such as skin, hair and eye color, height, body shape, type of blood, sex etc. The sex of the unborn child is determined by the type of chromosomes contributed by the male partner. For example, if a sperm carrying an X chromosome fertilizes the egg, the baby is a girl (XX), whereas the sperm carrying a Y chromosome fertilizes the egg, the baby is a boy (XY).

The lower part of the uterus is narrow and is called the cervix with an opening in its tip. The cervix projects into the vagina, creating the space between the vaginal walls and surface of the cervix called vaginal fornix. Cervical abnormalities are diagnosed clinically. Retention cysts of the cervix varying in size from a few millimeters to 4 cm. single or multiple are commonly diagnosed during routine sonogram. Cervical carcinoma is usually diagnosed clinically. About 4" in length the vagina runs from the cervix between the bladder and rectum. The upper broad end of the uterus opens on either side into two long tubes, called the fallopian tubes varying from 7 to 12 cm. in length, each ending in a funnel-shaped opening guarded by five finger-like projections. The cavity of the uterus is a potential space only, the anterior and posterior walls being normally in contact. The cavity of the body is triangular in shape 1" wide at the fundus and 1.5" long. The cavity of cervix is 1" long, and is spindle-shaped. The whole length of the uterine cavity is thus 2.5". The virgin uterus weighs about 42 gm. The measurement and the weight of uterus of a pregnant woman is slightly more than a virgin uterus. During pregnancy the uterus enlarges in order to contain the rapidly growing ovum inside it. At the beginning of pregnancy it is an organ measuring 3 by 2 by 1 inches. At the end of pregnancy it measures about 12 by 9 by 8 inches and its weight also increases from 45 to about 1000 gm. All the component tissues of the uterus share in this growth – the serous, muscular, mucous layers, the blood vessels, nerves and lymphatic.

The External Genitalia: The lower end of the vagina lies at the level of the hymen and of the introitus vagina, surrounded at this point by the erectile tissue of the bulb. The external organs of generation are generally called as vulva. The name and relative position of female external genital organs are Prepuce of clitoris, vestibule (anterior part), orifice of the vagina, vestbular fossa, glans clitoridis, frenulum, labium majus, Labium minus, orifice of the urethra and anus.

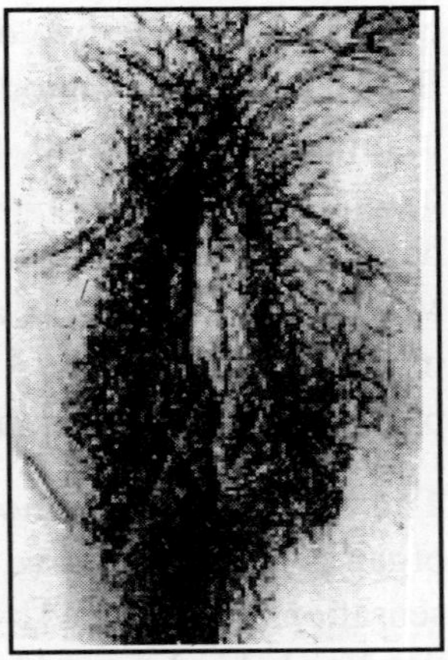

Female Genital Organ (outer View)

The Mons Pubis: Which is the only part of the genital organs visible when the woman is in the upright posture, which is a cushion of fat in front of the pubic symphysis, covered (after puberty) with curly hair. The mons pubis is

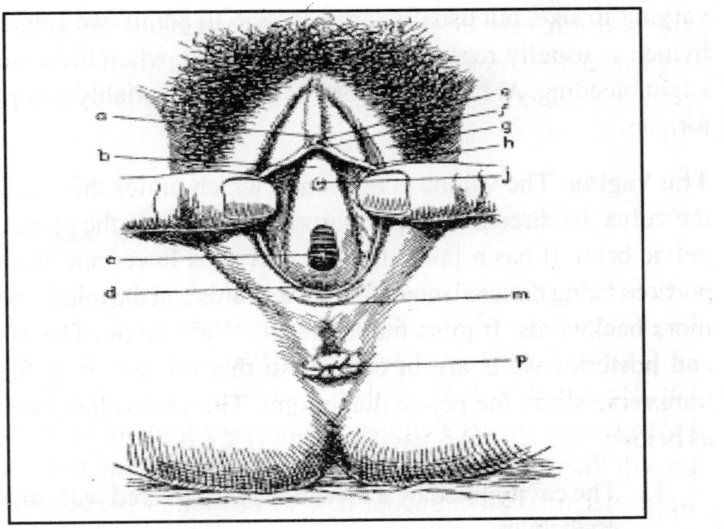

Female External Genital Organs

a. Prepuce of the clitoris b. Vestibule-anterior part c. Oriface of the vagina d. Vestibular fossa e. Glans Clitoris f. Labium majus h. Labium minus j. Oriface of the urethra m. posterior commissure p. Anus continued into the two outer lips of the vulva – the labia majora. Between the labia majora, in the case of most virgins there are two triangular folds of soft, smooth, moist skin - the labia minora or nymphae, which meet as the prepuce of the clitoris. They have no hair, are well supplied with sebaceous and sweat glands. The Vestibule is the smooth, almond-shaped area bounded by the labia minor on the both side. At its apex is the clitoris, and in the center is perforated by the urethra and the vagina..

The Clitoris is the homologue of the penis in the male. The whole organ is highly sensitive and is regarded as seat of the voluptuous sensations experienced by the female during coitus. Vaginal Orifice lies just behind the orifice of the urethra usually bounded by the hymen. In the virgin it is more or less closed by the hymen, and is completely hidden by the labia minora. Hymen is a circular fold of connective tissue covered with skin – like that of the vagina. It closes in the orifice of the vagina in the virgin leaving an aperture varying in size, but usually large enough to admit one finger. The hymen is usually ruptured at the first coitus, when there may be slight bleeding. At the first labor it is almost invariably completely torn up.

The Vagina: The vagina is the canal, which unites the uterus and the vulva. Its direction is approximately parallel to the plane of the pelvic brim. It has a faint sigmoid curve, its lower and the upper portions being directed more directly upwards and the middle portion more backwards. It joins the uterus at a right angle. The anterior and posterior walls are in contact so that on section it forms a transverse slit in the pelvic diaphragm. The vagina has four coats as below:

1. The cavity lined by a modified skin covered with stratified epithelium.
2. Below the epithelial layer is another layer of connective tissue, which passes towards the surface in the form of papillae.

3. The muscular layer, with its subdivision into an inner circular and outer longitudinal layer.

4. The outermost layer is the connective tissue sheath containing large plexus of veins and free blood supply.

The Penis: Penis is the male genital organ that serves a dual function of erection and as a route of excretion of urine and semen. It is composed of three cylindrical structures of cavernous – the two corpora cavernosa are the main erectile structures. The blood supply to the penis is primarily is made through arteries at the base of the penis, which supply blood to the skin and glans of the penis. Until recently, it was felt that psychological factors cause male

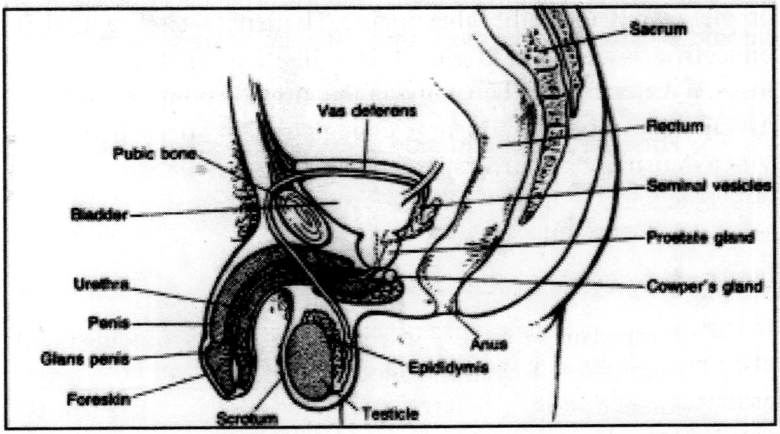

impotence. However, studies have revealed that a majority of the cases of impotence have organic causes. Subsequent studies have shown that vasculogenic impotence due to poor arterial inflow into the penis is one of the most frequent causes for erectile failure. Venogenic impotence is caused due to venous leakage of blood in the penis. The causes of the impotence are as following:

* Vasculogenic 37.5%

* Diabetes mellitus	20%
* Psychogenic	11.7%
* Neurogenic	6.7%
* Malegnancy	5.8%
* Testoterone and Trauma	3.3%
* Other causes	11.7%.

Ovary: Ovary has 1.5 inch length, 0.75 inch breadth and thickness resembles the egg of a pigeon in appearance are almond-shaped flattened bodies. It is connected with the base of the uterus by means of ligament tightly attached to the fallopian tubes. Poly-cystic ovary disease is a complex endocrine disturbance resulting from chronic in-ovulation. The most common symptoms are the following:

- Amenorrhea (Causing menstruation disorders).
- Hirsutism (accumulation of excess superfluous hair on the body).
- Obesity and infertility.
- Poly-cystic ovarian diseases.
- Formation of cysts e.g. functional cysts, follicular cyst, corpus-luted cyst and theca-luteal cysts.
- Ovarian remnant syndrome (causing pelvic inflammatory disease or tumor).
- Par-ovarian cysts and post-menopausal adnexal cysts.
- Endometriosis (presence of functioning endometrial tissue outside the uterus).

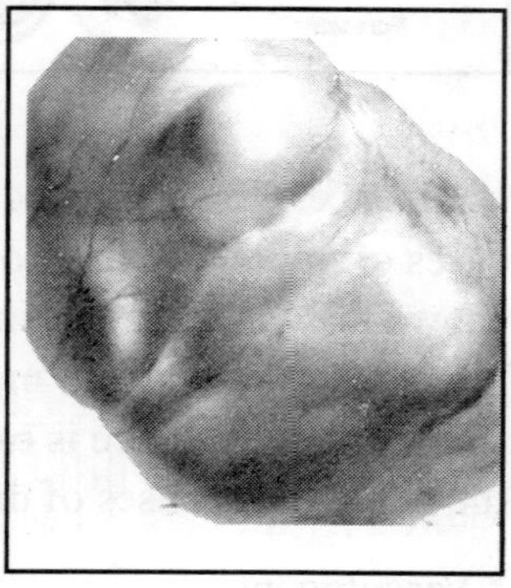

- Torsion of the ovary associated with cysts or tumors and ovary cancer.
- Epithelial tumors are harmful lesions, which need immediate treatment.
- Pelvic inflammatory disease is a common condition that is increasing in frequency due to diseased ovary. It is usually bilateral and caused by sexually transmitted diseases causing pain, fever and vaginal discharge. Ultrasound and Laproscopy are popular methods to detect ovarian disorders.

Abdomen and Liver: Abdomen is the seat of the functioning of all body organs. The liver is the largest organ in the human body weighing approximately 1500 gm. in the adult. The liver lies in the right upper portion of the abdomen, suspended from the right hemi-diaphragm. It can be divided into three lobes: the right, left and candate lobes. The right lobe of the liver is separated from left by the main lobar fissure. The left inter-segmental fissure divides the left lobe into medical and lateral segments. The candate lobe is situated on the posterior aspect of the liver. Liver has many important functions to perform, for it is great chemical laboratory of your body. The liver can be affected by a number of serious disorders, such as virus infections, parasites, disturbed circulation, stone formation in the bile duct, injuries due to poisonous substance and various kinds of tumors. Most of the foods we eat are stored in the liver; after having been digested and absorbed from the gastro-intestinal tract.

A vast network of tiny blood vessels arises from stomach, small bowel and spleen which in turn flow into the liver. Food materials from the digestive tract are able to reach the liver cells, where they are chemically changed and stored. These energy foods and vitamins stored in the liver are stock piled, which are needed by muscles, bones, nerve and other tissues. The various abnormalities of liver are liver cyst, jaundice, hepatitis, infections, serum, toxic and amoebic, fatty liver, cirrhosis of the liver and cancer of the liver described briefly as below:

- **Jaundice**: A disease marred by a yellow discoloration in the skin or in the whitest of the eyes. To treat jaundice, one must first find the cause of the jaundice. If the trouble is due to some parasite such as malaria parasite, proper medication may bring the condition under control. If the jaundice is due to presence of a stone or other obstruction, surgery will be needed for relief and cure.
- **Hepatitis**: An acute inflammation of liner caused by infectious or tonic agent. The skin may be discolored and the whites of the eye turn yellow. Various substances and organisms may be responsible for hepatitis, including germs, viruses, toxic agents and many other substances.
- **Infectious hepatitis**: Often occurs in the epidermis due to certain viruses spread mainly by contaminated food or water.
- **Fatty liver**: It is due to excessive amount of fat being deposited in the liver cells, which occur most frequently in overweight persons or due to excessive intake of food, particularly fat.
- **Cancer:** May arise in almost any organ of the body. When it begins in stomach or large bowel, the liver may soon be involved.

The Gall Bladder and Pancreatitis: The Gall Bladder is a small, pear-shaped, muscular organ closely attached to the under surface of the liver. The size and shape of normal gall-bladder (usually its transverse diameter exceeds 5 cm. vary widely in individual patients. The disorders of gall bladder include signs and symptoms of acute or chronic cholecystitis and jaundice. Cancer sometimes occurs in gall bladder. In as much as a person can live quite well without the gall bladder, it is wise to have diseased organ removed to avoid the risk of serious complications. Pancreas is an important gland situated below the lever, which produces strong digestive juices necessary for assimilation of food. Pancreatitis means inflammation of the organs – which may be mild or very severe. The treatments vary according to the seriousness of the condition. Avoid taking alcohol in any form, for this may only aggravate the condition. Avoid stress as far as possible.

The Urinary Tract: The human body is a living engine, which burns fuel. – the food and requires a constant supply of oxygen as well as water and various chemical substances, which provide energy to the organs of the body, and for repairing the damaged tissues constantly, keeping check on all these living cells and chemicals are two remarkable organs – kidneys.

Normally, the body filters about 300 liters of fluid each day leaving approximately one liter of urine to be excreted from the body. As the urine flows down the tiny tubules towards the center of kidney, it is finally collected in the renal pelvic, from there it finds its way down through the uterus to the bladder, where it remains until it is eliminated from the body. The common disorders of the urinary tract are following:

- Kidney stones.
- Poly-cystic disease (which begins before birth).
- Bright's disease (nephritis).
- Cancer of the urinary tract.
- Hydronephrosis.
- Kidney infection.
- Prostate gland.
- Tuberculosis of kidney.
- Urethritis (inflammation).
- Uraemia (toxic condition associated with kidney failure).

2

Disorders Before Conceiving

Vericose veins

Enlarged superficial veins usually into and around the legs due to increased pressure on the veins, which cause to lose the elasticity and become elongated. Varicose veins look like a bluish snake-like appearance.

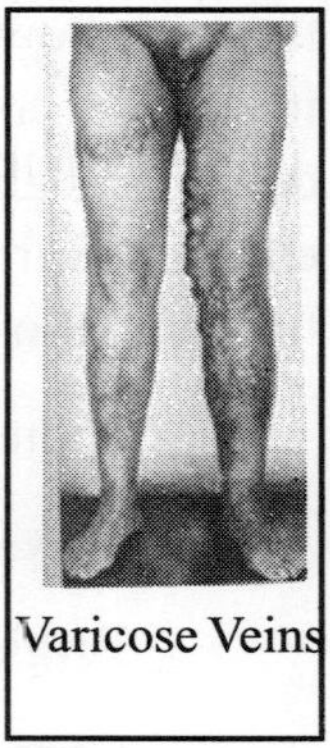

Varicose Veins

As the blood returns to the heart it passes through special thin-walled channels called veins. These vessels are easily distended and swell as the blood builds up behind it. Blood flows from the head and upper chest flows downward towards the heart. On the other hand, blood coming from the lower extremities must flow upward. To make it possible nature has provided valves in the veins so that blood can flow only towards the heart, never in other direction. Constipation, smoking and hot baths are all contributory factors to varicose veins.

The valves in the varicose veins in the legs (especially around the ankles and valves) and thighs are incompetent to prevent a backflow of blood resulting in stagnation followed by swelling, pain, inflammation or phlebitis. When the person suffering from varicose veins has been standing for a long time usually lead to reduced blood supply to the muscles. Varicose veins seem to run in families. This ailment is more frequent in pregnancy and obesity due to increased pressure in the pelvis or abdomen region, which slow the flow of blood to the heart from the lower extremities. The following measures are suggested to treat varicose veins:

- Check weight as every extra amount added to the weight increases the pressure on venous circulation.
- Blood sugar should remain within prescribed limits.
- Avoid prolonged standing.
- Wear comfortable padded low-heel shoes.
- Wear varicose vein stockings available at a chemist or surgical store.
- A hot and cold footbath before bed time improves circulation, prevents varicosities and helps to heal.
- Walking or jogging in water (in a swimming pool) is very helpful to relieve varicose veins.
- Vitamin C strengthens vein walls (Recommended dose 2,000 to 3000 mg daily).
- Rosemary tea with honey and elderflower tea are old-fashioned remedies to aid the circulation.
- Raise the legs several times a day and sleep with the foot of the bed raised six to eight inches higher than the head side.
- Massage the legs gently but do not scratch varicose veins because the varicose ulcers may result in from a sore place and can be very unpleasant. Excellent massage oils for varicose veins are olive oil, sweet almond oil, Essential oils of cypress, calendula, rosemary and lavender.

The signs of trouble include swelling along the course of the veins, followed by muscle cramps and a tired feeling of legs behind the knees. Sometimes, the skin over the lower part of the leg may break down forming a large, ugly painful ulcer. Surgery is the best treatment, especially when the large veins of the legs and thighs are involved. However, regular practice of yoga relieves varicose veins and cramps.

Vaginal Infections

Very common in females of every age when a yellowish discharge from vagina accompanied by itching can be due to fungal or bacterial infection. Candid V6/V3 is used for treating fungal infection. For bacterial infection certain other medicines as recommended by a doctor are useful. Get a high vaginal swab for culture sensitivity done. There is great need of cleanliness of genital area during pregnancy. The following are some of the common warning signs during pregnancy:

Warning Signs	Possible Problems
Vaginal bleeding	* Miscarriage
	* Placenta previa
	* Premature labor
Abdominal pain	* Ectopic pregnancy
	*Premature labor contractions
Leakage of fluid from vagina	* Rupture of membranes
Puffiness or swelling of face, hands and feet	* Preeclampsia (toxemia)
Severe/ persistent headache	* Pre-eclampsia (toxemia)
Pain/ burning while urinating	* Urinary tract infection
	* Sexually transmitted disease

Irritating vaginal discharge, soreness or itching	* Urinary tract infection * Sexually transmitted disease
Nausea or vomiting	* Hyperemesis gravidarum
Loose vaginal muscles	*Infection

Loose vaginal muscle has ruined many happy marriages. Remember, One cannot prove that women with loose vaginal muscles are not virgin, nor these muscles will be an hindrance in satisfying the male partner. Practice of yoga exercises help relieve. Vajroli Mudra is a yogic postures, which helps to tighten and strengthen loose vaginal muscles, relieve the disorders of pelvic region and strengthen all sex organs among both sexes. This exercise strengthens the anterior and posterior parts of the pubic muscles. A pregnant woman should do about 5 to 6 rounds of this posture daily strictly in consultation with a doctor.

To practice Vajroli Mudra, sit in Padma Asana (Lotus Pose) or any comfortable meditative asana. Place hands on knees, close eyes, feel relax and breathe through nose. After a deep inhalation, hold breath and try to draw the sexual organs upward by pulling and tensing the lower abdomen contracting the pelvic muscles as if one has an urge to pass urine but wishes to hold one for some time. Now exhale, relax and repeat the posture. This posture also helps those suffering from premature ejaculation and delay climaxing (orgasm) when involved in intercourse.

No periods due to closed hymen

Sexually well-developed teenage females sometimes do not have menses despite good health, although they feel periodic pains for few days every month besides having pain in the lower belly during these days. In few cases an ultrasound report showed a completely closed hymen. Surgical operation helps to start normal periods. Consult a doctor.

Marriage in blood relation

Marriage between blood relations is genetically unhealthy as both father and mother may carry the same type of unhealthy genes, which could intensify the unhealthy manifestation in the offspring. Here is an example of a couple both were closely related having blood relation. Their first baby was mentally retarded. They had an abnormal second baby. The third, a premature died at birth. The fourth also premature was, too, far from normal.

Duration of having sex

It depends upon the couples to involve into a pattern to suit their moods and needs. The frequency of the relationship varies from couple to couple. Some need sex everyday, others once or twice a month even in their early stage of marriage. With increasing age there is decline in sex in most of the couples. During pregnancy, frequent sex is not advisable and a couple must seek advice of a gynecologist. In case of problem pregnancy, better avoid sex as far as possible. In case of blood spots do not indulge in sex, this may lead to abortion.

Honeymoon urethritis

Over enthusiastic love making, excessive handling of clitoris during foreplay and frequent intercourse lead to severe inflammation of the urethral opening resulting in honeymoon urethritis. If the vagina has become infected or the infection is severe, pus cells pass into the bladder. Consult a doctor immediately fir the treatment.

Breast sucking

Sucking of breast by the husband is not harmful. If your husband wishes to suck the breasts, he should not be discouraged. This is natural and healthy exercise for the nipples and the breasts.

Natural contraceptive methods

Various contraceptive methods for the family planning are of three types as described below:

- **Coitus interrupts**: This is a unreliable and unhealthy method of contraception usually practiced by traditional couples in which the sex act is interrupted at the time of male ejaculation and the male organ is quickly withdrawn out of the vagina before the semen discharged out. However, long-term practice of coitus interrupts can cause pelvic congestion with the formation of ovarian cysts in the female.
- **Rhythm method**: This method follows the natural ovulation pattern in women, which happens once a month on the 14th day of the cycle (immediately before and after this day are the most fertile days for ovulation). However, the days following the menses and preceding the next period are the least fertile. The ovum is capable of getting fertilized for two or three days after its liberation as the discharged sperms remain vital for three or four days in the upper regions of the female genital tract. If the intercourse is avoided during ovulation and three to four days before and after, the chances of conception are minimal. The husband's cooperation is very necessary to avoid having sex for over a week in the mid cycle or use a condom during this period.
- **Lactating the baby**: In many women, during total lactation, ovulation stops and menses do not take place. During this period a woman cannot conceive or has very low fertility. This method, too, is not hundred percent reliable as there are instances, despite lactation, the woman conceives even before menstruation restart. In some cases, menstruation and ovulation commence within three months. The early restart of sex brings on quicker menstruation and ovulation due to hormonal effect on the system with breast milk decreasing.
- **Vasectomy and tubectomy**: Sterilizing the male or the female is the best way for permanent stop to birth of a

child. In males the operation is called Vasectomy in which the ducts (vas) carrying the sperms from the testes to the urethra in the penis is cut on both sides and tied beneath the skin of the scrotum. This operation is usually100% successful. Vasectomy has no fears about loss of libido, difficulty to perform the sex act and general debilitating effects. Vasectomy if performed un-hygienically can produce infection in the internal genital organs. In few cases the operation causes minor nerve pain during erection. In female the operation is known as Tubectomy in which the fallopian tubes on either side are cut and ligatured. The operation is performed easily, even a week after the delivery of child when the uterus is still high up in position and tubes are easy to ligature. The operation is performed by Laproscopy technique by a pencil like instrument fitted with microscope (micro surgery) with hardly an inch long cut into the abdomen.

Displacement of uterus

The uterus or the womb is slung in the pelvic cavity and has sufficient movement in all directions. However, its natural position is upwards and forwards between the bladder and rectum. Displacement of uterus occurs because of several reasons and is usually accompanied by inflammation. The downward displacement of uterus is known as pro-lapse. In this condition the uterus slips downwards in the space between bladder and rectum. This condition is more common in overweight or too weak women.

The disorder is frequent in women having repeated deliveries. The uterus gets distend during pregnancy when the fetus grows. The muscles supporting the uterus become to week to bear the burden of the growing child in it. After the delivery of child the uterus and surrounding muscles lacks the former shape and the size. The symptom, which indicate displacement of the uterus include backache or headache and heaviness in the bowels. Nerve centers are badly affected due to the displacement of uterus. The patient feels irritable and depressed. Doctors generally advise surgical interference for the treatment.

All external or internal muscles of the body if become loose, their tone and strength start malfunctioning resulting in such ailment. Inactive muscles may also acquire extra coats of fat and become unserviceable. Lack of proper exercise, acquisition of a coat of fat, deposition of morbid matter in the body and an inadequate diet lacking in essential vitamins and mineral substances can lead to weakness of the muscles of the body. A healthy woman doesn't experience any difficulty in childbirth and there are no complications even afterwards. Remember, antenatal care and proper diet can ward off the danger of displacement of uterus. If the patient is weak and old, it could take long to put her back in shape. The following natural steps are recommended:

- Have good diet containing enough fruits, milk and green vegetables.
- Rest and relaxation in the bed drain out tension from the body.
- Have a regular exercise plan designed to tone up the muscles supporting the uterus. Also seek advice of a naturopath doctor.
- Rub the parts immersed in water vigorously while having Hip Bath.
- Keep a hard pillow under the buttocks instead of under the head. This will help the uterus to return to its initial position.
- Lie on the floor with your knees touching your breast, which help the uterus to resume its normal position.
- Lie down after a meal with a pillow under your back.

Premature ejaculation

It is a malfunctioning due to psychological reasons generally found in males who are sexually more aroused than the females, who need a bit of foreplay to be ready for the intercourse. Too much anticipation of the sex act, too much of excitement can lead to premature ejaculation giving a feeling of failure or lack of fulfillment, which should follow the act of sexual intercourse. The following are natural ways to treat premature ejaculation:

- Apply Mud Pack on pubes before sleep at night.
- Kegal Exercise: Squeeze the muscles in the anal area as if you are trying to stop the flow of urine. This exercise strengthens the muscles of all genital organs, the urethra (urinary tube) and the rectum. A regular practice will help you to control over ejaculation.
- Self-stimulation: If you want to learn to slow your minutes' ejaculation reflex for four to six times during each session, masturbate three to four times a week, just bringing you close to orgasm but without ejaculating.
- Scrotal Pull Technique: During self-stimulation try practicing to pull down on your scrotal sac before you reach the point of no return. During sex, you can do it yourself or seek the help of your partner.
- Press the area on your perineum, the space between the anus and the back of the scrotum, which stimulates the prostate – the gland that supplies the fluid for semen during ejaculation. Pressing on this spot when you are highly aroused helps block the ejaculatory reflex and can be quite pleasurable and delays ejaculation. Press on it firmly and rhythmically at any point on the area during sex after you have achieved a maximum erection.
- Mix in equal quantity seeds of 'Lajwanti' and sugar and take with the milk in the morning.
- Avoid constipation and digestion disorders.

Male impotence

Impotence (sexual weakness) is the inability to perform sex - it may be partial or complete, temporary or permanent. Impotence can be in two categories: as a result of organic reasons or psychological reasons as described below:

Organic impotence: is caused by the following reasons:

- Lesions of the external genitalia such as a tight foreskin.
- Disturbances of endocrine glands, such as diminished activity of the gonads, thyroid glands or pituitary glands.
- Diseases of the central nervous system.
- Severe disturbance of health.
- Diabetes plays an adverse effect in this case.

In case of treatment of impotency due to organic factors, deal with the disease caused it.

Psychological impotence: is caused by the following factors:

- Ignorance about sex.
- Fear.
- Weak-ness or abnormality of sexual desire.

The psychological treatment of impotence is to find the true reason and realize what has caused it. Treatment for impotency includes the following:

- The best remedy for impotence is a healthy diet and exercise.
- A wet pack (dipped in cold water) on the spine can help body to energize and strengthen the nervous system. Lie naked on the bed so that the wet bandage remains in constant touch with the spine.

- Drink plenty of water in a day to draw away all the morbid matter that has been poisoning the body system.
- Dry in the shade tender, seedless pods of Acacia and mix with the equal weight of Brown sugar. Take with the milk. Alternatively, tender leaf-shoots of Banyan tree may be substituted for Acacia pods.

Frigidity in women

Frigidity is a condition in women, where she is unable to give herself sexually to male partner and enjoy sex usually due to the following reasons:

- Psychological fear.
- Wrong notions about sex.
- Physical incapacity.
- Hormonal and genital defects.
- Cultural taboos and social position.
- Intellectual upbringing and emotional status playing a significant role in female sexual behavior.
- Sexual indifferences (which is the major reason) or disliking for sex.
- Physicals causes such as inflamed vagina, a very rigid hymen, urinary problems or uterine infections.
- Displaced ovaries.

Nocturnal emission

Involuntary discharge of semen (the fluid produced by testicles in male) during sleep or nocturnal emission is one of the common disorders among youths or even in middle-age persons. Night emission among youngsters is generally due to excitement because of reading vulgar literature or seeing a motion picture having exciting scenes. The following treatments are recommended to get rid of this psychological disorder:

- Avoid thoughts of sex.
- Eat rich food.
- Have dinner three hours before sleep.
- Have evening walk followed by a bath.
- Go to the bed early, not later than 9 p.m.
- Application of a Mud Pack on pubes during sleep at night.
- Hot and cold hip bath.

Excessive sex

There are women who are extremely passionate and feel uncontrolled sex desire. They are constantly attracted towards opposite sex. This is often due to the following reasons:

- Deep sense of insecurity produced by neglect in childhood and adolescence.
- Genetically, some females are hyper-fertile and highly sexual.

Excessively sexual women need psychotherapy. Hormone therapy neutralizes the effect of estrogen by administering progesterone hormones help to large extent.

Painful intercourse

The disorder is also known as Dyspareunia, which may arise from muscular spasm of the vagina. Sometimes, there is a superficial ulceration following some injury and tissues are painful to the touch. Bladder infection is common in such cases, which may lead to further complications. Some of the causes of a painful intercourse are following:

- Tightness in the female genital area after a surgery. In such case usually tissues may have been drawn too tightly together.
- Pelvic inflammation may cause pain during intercourse.
- Nervous tension usually due to unconsciously afraid of pregnancy.
- Problems like body odors, halitosis etc.
- Lack of understanding on the part of male partner,
- May cause her pain during marital relations.

When urine escapes

This disorder of leakage of urine while laughing or carrying an heavy luggage is generally due to weakness of urethral opening or weak vaginal muscles sometimes as a result of repeated childbirths and prolonged labor. The overstretched urethral opening loses its elasticity. Sometimes, the urine escapes out with increased abdominal pressure due to short length of urethra in females.

Night discharge

Involuntary discharge during sleep or at night while dreaming is common among youths. Reading cheap and vulgar literature or seeing sexually exploiting movies and TV serials may lead to frequent night discharge during sleep. There is misconception in our country that semen is produced from blood. Semen in males is, in fact, the fluid produced by testicles and its production during intercourse or involuntary discharge during sleep is not much of a concern as the quacks have us believe. Those concerned by frequent night discharge should take a clean, healthy living. Sexual thoughts and rich foods should be completely avoided. Rich foods only disturb the digestive system. Dinner should be taken three hours before sleep. To cure night ejaculation, get up early in the morning. Sunbath has a curative effect. Go to bed early preferably with a mud- pack on the pubic area. This regimen is equally beneficial for hysteria patients, to treat menstrual irregularities and in case of frigidity in women.

Premarital sex

Premarital sex is uncommon in Indian males as well as females due to early marriages. Sex life starts with marriage in most of the cases. Women feel the risk of pregnancy and avoid premarital sex. When a female goes through an abortion, it has physical risks to health and can produce hemorrhage, rupture of uterus, pelvic infection and other serious complications to catch pelvic infection, vaginitis, urinary infection and risk of sexually transmitted diseases.

Sex after menopause

Menopause is not the end of sex life and a woman can continue normal sex for years after she has stopped her periods. Many women enjoy satisfying sexual partnership even in old age. There are numerous couples in 60s who are involved in active sex life. Sometimes, menopausal women face problems having sex due to severe dryness of genital organs with pain during intercourse. Lubricating creams or estrogen ointments help to prevent rapid atrophy of the vaginal mucosa.

3

Abnormalities of Genital Organs

Every female getting married or on way to become a mother should know about her genital organs and their abnormalities thoroughly. Most of the teenagers and newly weds feel hesitant to question about their genitals abnormalities, though their knowledge is essential for every one to make married life and pregnancy more enjoyable and also allay fears and misconception.

The Uterus: The womb is the compartment of female body in which a baby forms and grows till birth. It is also termed as uterus, a pear-shaped hollow thick walled muscular organ situated deep in the lower abdomen, placed between the bladder in front and the rectum behind. The uterus is usually of size 3"x2"x1" when in non-pregnant state and it stretches gradually in size to accommodate a fully formed baby. The lower part of the uterus is narrow and is called the cervix with an opening in its tip. The cervix projects into the vagina, creating the space between the vaginal walls and surface of the cervix also called vaginal fornix. The upper end of the uterus opens on either side into two long tubes, called the fallopian tubes varying from 7 cm. to 12 cm. in length, each ending in a funnel-shaped opening guarded by five finger-like projections called 'fimbria'.

The funnel-shaped opening lies close to the ovary on either side. The cavity of the uterus is a potential space only, the anterior and posterior walls being normally in contact. The cavity of the body is triangular in shape 1" wide at the fundus and 1.5" long. The cavity of cervix is 1" long, and is spindle-shaped. The whole length of the uterine cavity is thus 2.5". The virgin uterus weighs between 40 to 42 gm. The measurement and the weight of uterus of a pregnant woman is more than a virgin uterus. During pregnancy the uterus enlarges in order to contain the rapidly growing ovum inside it. At the beginning of pregnancy it is an organ measuring 3 by 2 by 1 inches. At the end of pregnancy it measures about 12 by 9 by 8 inches and its weight also increases from about 40 gm. to about 1000 gm. All the component tissues of the uterus share in this growth – the serous, muscular, mucous layers, the blood vessels, nerves and lymphatic.

External Genitals-Vagina: The external organs of generation are generally spoken of as the vulva. The name and relative position of female external genital organs are: Prepuce of the clitoris, Vestibule

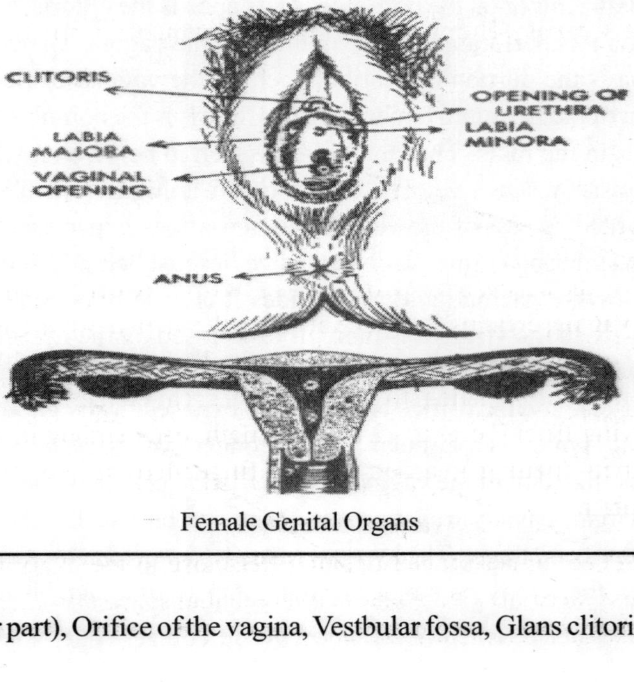

Female Genital Organs

(anterior part), Orifice of the vagina, Vestbular fossa, Glans clitoridis,

Frenulum, Labium majus, Labium minus, Orifice of the urethra, Posterior commissure and Anus. The Mons Pubis is the only part of the genital organs visible when the woman is in the upright posture, is a cushion of fat in front of the pubic symphysis, covered after puberty with more or less short curly hair. The mons pubis is continued in a backward direction into the two outer lip of vulva is called Labia Majora. Each labium majus has a lateral and a medial surface. The lateral is covered with the same short crisp hair that covers the mons. The medial surfaces, which are usually in opposition, are smoother and are devoid hair. Posteriorly the fat disappears from the labia, and they are just two folds of the skin that meet at the posterior commissure. Labia Minora lies between the labia majora, and in the case of most virgins visible only on drawing them apart, are two triangular folds of soft, smooth, moist skin.

The Vestibule: is the smooth, almond-shaped area bounded by the labia minor on the both side. At its apex is the clitoris, and in the center it is perforated by the urethra and the vagina. The vestibular fossa is the portion of vestibule behind the vaginal orifice and in front of the frenulum labiorum. The Clitoris is the homologue of the penis in the male. The small glans is rich in nerve endings, and is exquisitely sensitive. The whole organ is highly erectile, and is regarded as seat of the voluptuous sensations experienced by the female during coitus. Vaginal Orifice lies just behind the orifice of the urethra. Behind and at the sides it is usually bounded by the hymen. In the virgin it is more or less closed by the hymen, and is completely hidden by the labia minora. In many demales the hymen is absent, and the orifice is frequently exposed the by gaping of the labia. Hymen is a circular fold of connective tissue covered with skin – like that of the vagina. It closes in the orifice of the vagina in the virgin, leaving an aperture varying in size, but usually large enough to admit one finger. The hymen is usually ruptured at the first coitus, when there may be slight bleeding. At the first labor it is almost invariably completely torn up.

The Vagina: The vagina is the canal, which unites the uterus and the vulva. Its direction is approximately parallel to the plane of the pelvic brim. It has a faint sigmoid curve, its lower and the upper portions being directed more directly upwards and the middle portion more backwards. It joins the uterus at an angle, which is nearly a right angle. The anterior and posterior walls are in contact so that on section it forms a transverse slit in the pelvic diaphragm. The vagina has four coats as below:

- The cavity is lined by a modified skin covered with stratified epithelium.
- Below the epithelial layer is another layer of connective tissue, which passes towards the surface in the form of papillae, just as in the subcuticular layer of the skin.
- Next comes the muscular layer, with its subdivision into an inner circular and outer longitudinal layer.
- The outermost coat is the connective tissue sheath, which contains a large plexus of veins and very free blood supply.

Abnormalities of cervix and the vagina

Abnormalities of the cervix and vagina: Cervical abnormalities are diagnosed clinically. Retention cysts of the cervix varying in size from a few millimeters to 4 cm., single or multiple are commonly diagnosed during routine sonogram. Multiple cysts may be a cause of benign enlargement of the cervix. Cervical carcinoma is usually diagnosed clinically. The vagina, having four inches length runs anteriorly and caudally from the cervix between the bladder and rectum. Garner's duct cysts most common cystic lesions of the vagina are mesonephric duct remnants that form single or multiple cysts along the lateral wall of the vagina. Solid masses of the vagina are rare but common congenital abnormalities of the female genitract. As in carcinoma of cervix, sonogram is not used for diagnosis of the caranoma of the vagina.

How pregnancy develops?

Abdomen and Liver: Abdomen is the seat of the functioning of all body organs. The liver is the largest organ in the human body weighing approximately 1500 gm. in the adult. The liver lies in the right upper quardrant of the abdomen, suspended from the right hemidiaphragm. It can be divided into three lobes-the right, left and candate lobes. The right lobe of the liver is separated from left by the main lobar fissure. The left inter-segmental fissure divides the left lobe into medical and lateral segments. The candate lobe is situated on the posterior aspect of the liver. Your liver has many important functions to perform, for it is great chemical laboratory of your body. The liver can be affected by a number of serious disorders such as virus infections, parasites, disturbances of the circulation, stone formation in the bile duct, injuries due to poisonous substance and various kinds of tumors. Most of the foods we eat are stored in the liver; after having been digested and absorbed from the gastro-intestinal tract.

A vast network of tiny blood vessels arises from stomach, small bowel and spleen which in turn flow into the liver. Food materials from the digestive tract are able to reach the liver cells, where they are chemically changed and stored. These energy foods and vitamins stored in the liver are stock piled, which are needed by muscles, bones, nerve and other tissues. The various abnormalities of liver are liver cyst, jaundice, hepatitis, infections, serum, toxic and amoebic, fatty liver, cirrhosis of the liver and cancer of the liver Jaundice is a disease marred by a yellow discoloration in the skin or in the whitest of the eyes. To treat jaundice, one must first find the cause of the jaundice. If the trouble is due to some parasite such as malaria parasite, proper medication may bring the condition under control. If the jaundice is due to presence of a stone or other obstruction, surgery will be needed for relief and cure. Hepatitis is an acute inflammation of liner caused by infectious or tonic agent. The skin may be discolored and the whites of the eye turn yellow.

Various substances and organisms may be responsible for hepatitis, including germs, viruses, toxic agents and many other substances. Infectious hepatitis often occurs in the epidemis due to certain viruses spread mainly by contaminated food or water. Fatty liver is due to excessive amount of fat being deposited in the liver cells, which occur most frequently in overweight persons or due to excessive intake of food, particularly fat. Cancer may arise in almost any organ of the body. When it begins in stomach or large bowel, the liver may soon be involved.

4

Methods Of Family Planning

After marriage, a woman should know how to plan an ideal family and should be familiar with the various methods of family planning. Some of the prominent methods are condom for men, condom for women, use of diaphragm (rubber lid with a spring margin that closes the female cervix), cervical thimble-shaped cap (to be pushed into the vagina to cover the cervix), sponges and pessaries, vaginal tablets and creams, intra-uterine device, intra-cervical device, vaginal rings, oral contraceptives and natural contraceptives.

Birth control is also known as contraception, which refers to prevent fertilization-the union of the sperms and egg produced by ovaries. Most of the newly married couples want to know about the family planning techniques. Birth control is important in the following cases:

- When a woman is in poor state of health. She should try to control pregnancy until she is healthy enough to face the strain due to pregnancy and childbirth.
- When couples have a desire for children but want to space them out.
- If there have been previous Cesarean section deliveries a couple of times.

Following are various most widely used methods of birth control:

Abstinence

It is a truly safe method of birth control in which the semen ejaculated near the entrance of vagina without having had actual intercourse. In certain cases the ejaculated semen may come into contact with a virginal hymen and gain access to the vagina and reaches to the uterus. Some marriages were able to survive with this method.

Rhythm method

There is certain period every month when a woman is not likely to become pregnant. A woman in childbearing age sheds an egg from her ovary every month around the 14th day after the onset of her menstruation (with a regular 28 day interval) between the menstrual periods. She might ovulate between 12th to 16th days. The sperm can live for at least two days within the Fallopian tubes, the place at which fertilization takes place. Thus a woman is more likely to become pregnant in case of sexual contact during this period. This method is about 85-90% effective.

Coitus interruptus

This is one of the oldest methods of birth control if the male partner has proper control over the withdrawal of his organ and the other partner has no objection to this practice, as some women reach a climax when their male partner ejaculates. It is not a 100% safe method of birth control, as in few cases part of the semen ejaculated from male organ may remain deposited on the female organ. Males who suffer from premature ejaculation usually have poor control over the ejaculation. This method of birth control is not recommended as a regular practice as a man has a great need for complete sexual act once started.

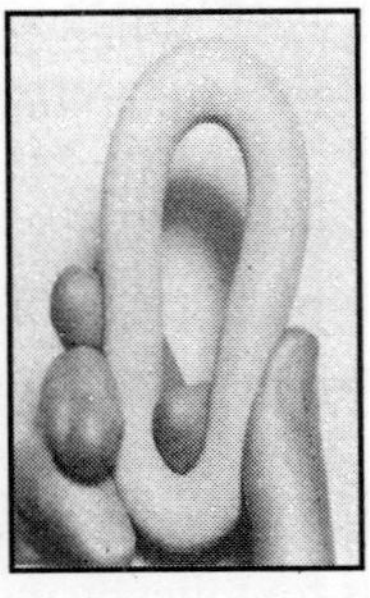

Condom

A thin latex sheath placed on the male organ to collect ejaculation of the semen. This is a frequently used safe method for birth control. The condom is discarded and thrown after single use. Most of the couples complain of lack of enjoyment during sexual act when a condom is used and is not preferred due to the following reasons:

1. Decrease sensation when used.
2. Interrupt lovemaking when put on.
3. It may break while in use.
4. It may leak due to a manufacturing defect or expiry.
5. It may burst when in use or slip off after orgasm before removing.

Precaution: In case of leakage, the woman should immediately place one or two contraceptive suppositories or contraceptive jelly or foam deep into her vaginal canal. Avoid douching.

Douches

It is cleansing of vaginal canal by use of a syringe and stream of water. It is one of the poorest methods because it is not possible to flush out completely by douching and some of the sperms in the folds of the vagina may penetrate into the cervix.

Diaphragm

It is a circular rubber device that fits tightly in the vagina completely covering the cervix. A gynecologist may suggest the correct size of diaphragm after examination. The diaphragm can be inserted while standing or lying on the back or in sitting position as one sits for toilet by inserting

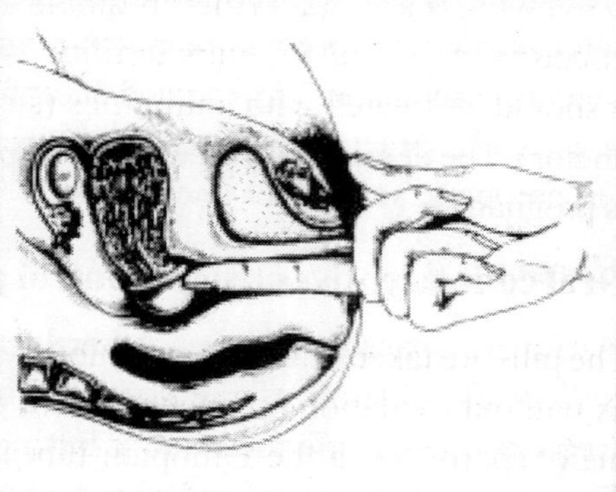

Fixing Cervical Cap

fingers. The front end of the diaphragm will be tucked in back of the pubic bone. The diaphragm is removed the next morning or about five hours after termination of relations.

Contraceptive jellies, foams and creams

They are highly effective products in destroying sperm within the vagina. These are inserted into the vagina an hours before the intercourse. You may follow the instructions mentioned on the wrapper before use.

Intrauterine devices (IUDs)

A plastic or plastic-metal object inserted by the gynecologist into the uterine cavity. It is 98% effective device. The cervix is dilated, usually during a menstrual period and the device is pushed into the uterine cavity. However, women feel mild discomfort. The device blocks the entrance of the sperm into the Fallopian tube where fertilization takes place. The device is usually changed after three years. The IUD should not be inserted or removed if inserted in case of the following conditions such as the woman has heavy menstrual periods or bleeding in between the periods, has fibroid tumors, have extremely painful menstruation, suffers from lower abdominal cramps and there is cervical infection. However, a woman who has not borne any children should avoid wearing an IUD as an infection may result in future fertility. In case of a uterine infection, it should be treated with antibiotics (strictly as per the advice of a doctor). The device should be removed promptly in case the woman is pregnant.

Oral contraceptives (Birth control pills)

The pills are taken orally. They inhibit ovulation or formation of egg, as without ovulation pregnancy is not possible regardless of how many sperm reach the Fallopian tubes. Each tablet contains two female hormones: estrogen and progesterone. These pills are 100% effective and should be taken strictly according to the advice of your doctor. It eliminates any disagreeable contraceptive odor. Sometimes, complications as below may arise while taking the birth control pills:

1. A feeling of headaches and nausea.
2. A bloated feeling with some weight gain due to fluid retention.
3. Swelling and tenderness in the breasts may develop.
4. Inflammation of the veins in the legs (known as plebitis).

Avoid using oral contraceptives in case of obese women, women having chronically high blood pressure, if suffering from liver disorder, in case of heavy smokers, if suffering from varicose veins or phlebitis, heavy smokers, in older women, when suffering from fibroids of the uterus, women having breast tumor or have cystic disease of the breasts and family history of breast disorders.

Surgical birth control

An incision is made in the lower abdomen, the tubes are grasped with a forceps and tied or cut in their middle portion or are cauterized with an electric cautery.

Laparoscope

This metal instrument is inserted through incision in the navel through which the gynecologist looks in the abdomen and applies the cautery to the Fallopian tubes. It is a 100% effective method for birth control.

Vasectomy

It is a technique for cutting the vas deferens, thereby making the male infertile. In case the couple has many children and the husband wishes to spare the wife the discomfort of surgery. However, cutting the vas in no way interferes with a man's potency or ability to have or enjoy sex.

Severe labor pains

Prolonged Labor: A labor that lasts longer than 24 hours is called a prolonged labor. The more important is phase of labor in which there are reasons for slow progress and rate of cervical dilation. A prolonged labor process can discourage, exhaust and emotionally drain or may turn to complication an expectant mother. Do not become discouraged or depressed in case of a prolonged labor. The expectant mother should be nurtured with food or drink, bath and showers, walks and backrubs. Consult your doctor and try various methods to stimulate labor. Medical interventions are essential if labor prolongs more than 24 hours. Stimulate effective contractions with procedures such as stripping the membranes, administering an enema or giving drugs that ripen the cervix to induce labor. The following steps are advised in case of prolonged labor:

- Turn by changing position every 20 to 30 minutes encouraging the baby to turn to position taking advantage of gravity and movement.
- Stand or walk to try to align the baby's body with the entrance to the pelvis and pelvic flexibility.
- Do the pelvic rock, which may free the baby's head from the pelvis and allow it to turn to an anterior position.
- There is often severe back pain due to prolonged labor. To relieve back pain, prevent baby's head from pressing on your back, apply counter-pressure on your back, ask your partner for a back massage, use hot or cold pack on your low back during or between contractions, stand or sit in the shower and let the water spray on the painful area and use pain medications if necessary.

What is perineal massage?

Perineal massage is used to soften the tissue around the vagina and increase the elasticity of the perineum by taking advantage of the hormonal changes that loosen connective tissues in late pregnancy. It also encourages you to relax the pelvic floor muscles when there is pressure. Perineal massage helps to avoid episiotomy or severe pain during delivery. Massage the perineum daily for about six weeks before your due date. If you suffer from vaginitis, herpes or other vaginal problems, make sure to consult your doctor before beginning perineal massage as it could worsen the condition. Either you or your partner can do the massage. Be sure that your fingernails are short and hands are clean. If you are massaging yourself, massage before a mirror and look at your perineum so that you can see what you are doing.

Before you start massaging, lubricate your fingers well with oil or water-soluble jelly. Wheat-germ oil is best recommended for perineal massage because it contains high vitamin E contents. Do not use mineral oil or petroleum jelly. Rub enough oil or jelly into the perineum to allow your fingers to move smoothly over the tissues and lower vaginal walls. You can use your thumb if massaging yourself, whereas your male partner can use his index finger. Put the finger and the thumb well inside the vagina in a rhythmic U or sling-type movement to stretch the vaginal tissue, skin of the perineum and muscles surrounding the vagina. Massage not more than five minutes.

Bleeding after the childbirth

Mostly bleeding will occur after labor and delivery of baby. However, if you lose more than two cups of blood, you may be hemorrhaging (a steady flow of blood and symptoms of shock, rapid pulse, paleness, trembling, cold and sweating. If you suspect hemorrhage, massage the uterus firmly through the abdominal wall until it contracts and encourage the newly born baby to nurse besides massaging breast nipples. If the bleeding appears at the vaginal opening, pad the perineum with an ice pack and towels. Apply firm pressure.

5

Signs and Symptoms of Pregnancy & Abortion

Signs & symptoms of Pregnancy ?

- Stoppage of Menstruation (monthly bleeding known as periods).
- Laziness, heavy feeling, irritability and presence of physical disturbances.
- Morning sickness and vomiting from second month onwards, which usually stops in the fourth month, or in some cases continues throughout pregnancy period.
- Heaviness in breasts.
- Breast nipples get prominent and areola starts turning darker from pinkish.
- Tightening of abdomen after about four months.
- Pressure of the pregnant uterus on the urinary bladder.
- Genitals feel warmer due to more blood and congestion.
- Vagina remains excessive moist.
- The fetal movement starts usually in the fifth month onward.
- Vagina is usually hot and moist.
- Uterus rises above the pelvis when the pregnancy is

advanced.

- The movement of the fetus increases, feeling the limbs, head and neck of the fetus.
- Nausea and vomiting (start two weeks after the conception).
- Exhaustion and tiredness.
- Change of taste.
- Strong liking and disliking for certain foods.

Abortion

Loss or failure of early pregnancy in several forms: complete, incomplete, inevitable, missed, septic and threatened is known as Abortion.

Complete abortion: The termination of a pregnancy before the age of viability almost in 50% cases. It occurs at less than 20 weeks from the first day of the last normal menstrual period or involving a fetus of weight less than 500 gm.

Incomplete abortion: The spontaneous passage of some of the products of conception associated with uniform pregnancy loss.

Inevitable abortion: A pregnancy in which rupture of the membranes and/or cervical dilation take place during the first half of the pregnancy period.

Missed abortion: The retention of an failed intrauterine pregnancy detected by an ultrasound.

Septic abortion: A variant of an incomplete abortion due to infection.

Threatened abortion: An pregnancy where vaginal bleeding or uterine cramping occurs. 50-60% such pregnancies come in the category of complete abortion.

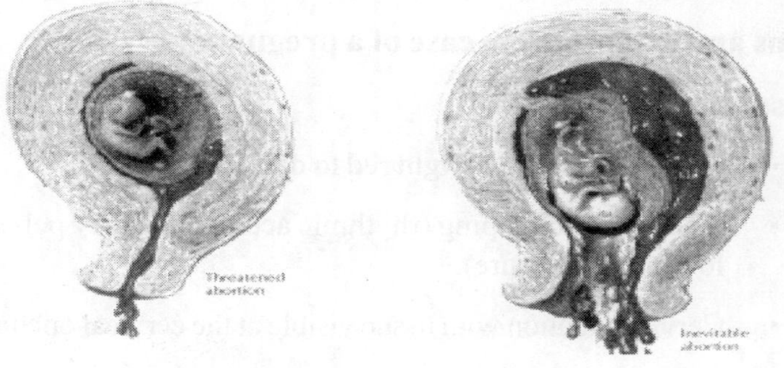

Threatened Abortion

Causes of abortion

There are several causes for an abortion. Some of the prominent causes are the following:

- Endocrine abnormalities (in 25-50% cases).
- Genetic factors (in 10-70% cases).
- Trisomy (in 40-50% cases).
- Monosomy (in 15-25% cases).
- Reproductive tract abnormalities (in 6-12% cases).
- Tripoidy and tetraploidy (in 5-15% cases).
- Abnormality of placenta.
- Effect of venereal diseases.
- Chronic cardiovascular disease and chronic renal disease.

- Diabetes mellitus.
- Environmental factors such as alcohol, anesthetic gases, effect of drugs, radiation, smoking and toxins.
- Other factors such as advanced maternal age, delayed fertilization, short interval between pregnancies.

Signs and symptoms in case of a pregnancy

These include the following:

- Vaginal bleeding (bright red to dark colored).
- Abdominal cramping (rhythmic accompanied by pelvic or low back pressure).
- Cervical dilation with tissue visible at the cervical openings.
- Severe vaginal hemorrhage.
- Cervical polyps and cervicitis.
- Urinary tract infection and lower abdominal discomfort.
- Loss of early symptoms such as fullness of breasts or morning sickness.
- Disseminated intra-vascular coagulopathy can occur when an intrauterine fetal demise in the second trimester has been retained beyond six weeks after the death of the fetus.

Specific measures

- Rh-negative mothers should be treated with Rh immune globulin after completion of the abortion, because ovulation may occur as early as two weeks after an abortion.
- After an abortion, control the bleeding, prevent infection and relieve pain.
- Ensure that all the products of the conception have been expelled from the uterus. If retained tissues are present

and cannot be rules out, curettage must be performed immediately.

- Septic abortion requires urgent and aggressive management. Antibiotics, fluid therapy and prompt evacuation of the uterus are indicated.
- If significant pain or bleeding persists, especially bleeding leading to hemo-dynamic alterations, evacuation of the uterus should be conducted.

Maternal disorders and their effect on the fetus

Disorder	Adverse effect
Toxemia of pregnancy:	Intra-uterine growth retardation, respiratory depression of the fetus due to use of sedatives and need for curtailment of pregnancy.
Antepartum hemorrhage:	Fetal and birth asphyxia, premature labor and anemia.
Polyhydramnios:	Anencephaly, high intestinal obstruction and ectopic pregnancy.
Oligohydramnios:	Bilateral renal agenesis or hypoplasia obstructive, obstructive uropathy, deformed limbs or face.
Rupture of membranes:	High risk of pneumonia in the baby.
Malnutrition:	Intrauterine growth retardation, anemia (iron deficiency).
Thyrotoxicosis:	Neonatal thyrotoxicosis and goiter.
Maternal diabetes:	Premature delivery, often by cesarean section, intrauterine death, early asymptomatic or symptomatic hypoglycemia.

Maternal infection:	Abortion, intrauterine death, fetal growth retardation, multisystem involvement such as hepatitis, meningoencephalitis, anemia, thrombocytopenia, microcephaly or hydrocephaly, congenital malformation with viral infections during the first trimester of pregnancy.

6

Types of Pregnancy

Radiological diagnosis of pregnancy: This is widely used method for the diagnosis of pregnancy. The main reasons for the employment of radiography are the following:

1. The diagnosis of pregnancy.
2. The demonstration of the fetus in relation to presentation and position, maturity, structural abnormalities and multiple pregnancy intra-uterine death.
3. The demonstration of the uterus with reference to hydramnios and placental situation when the placenta praevia is suspended.
4. Localization of fetal abdomen for the purpose of intra-uterine transfusion.
5. Demonstration of material pelvis and lumber spine including pelvimetry.

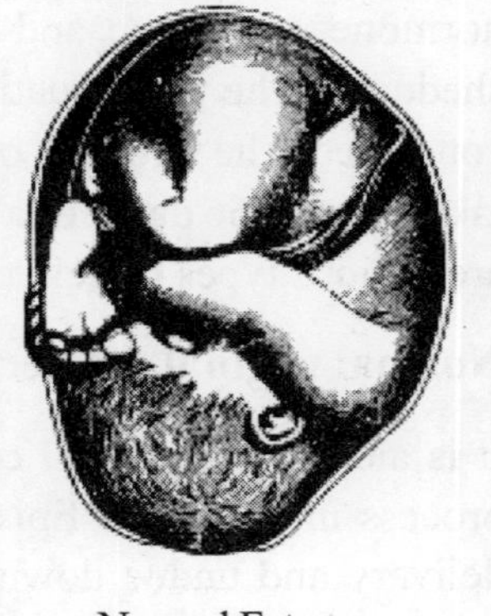

Normal Fetus

Radiological method of diagnosis should not be employed before the 28th week and are rarely necessary thereafter to find out the structural abnormalities and in twin pregnancy when one head is nearer the X-ray tube than other. To find out a multiple pregnancy, the demonstration of the uterus and placental situation, hydramnios and placenta praevia, tube shift method is employed in the following ways:

- Find out first view of the pelvic inlet demonstrated in contour in the antero-posterior projection. The X-ray tube is centered above the patient's pelvis, so that the central ray of the X-ray beam passes through about three inches behind the anterior border of symphysis pubis.
- The radiograph is taken with the patient lying on the left side in between the left loin to keep the lumber spine straight. The thighs are flexed 5 degree towards the abdomen and knees are flexed 90 degree.
- The radiograph to show the transverse diameter of the outlet and the sub-pubic angle is obtained by placing the patient in sitting position. The X-ray beam is directed vertically downwards so that it passes through the mid point of the line joining the two tuberosities.

The types of deliveries

Fertilization is the union of a mature ovum with a sperm. If sexual intercourse takes place within 12 to 24 hours of ovulation, then one of the thousands of sperms deposited in vagina unites with the ovum to fertilize it after traveling uterine cavity and reaching fallopian tube. Once the pregnancy has not established, the production of the hormones- estrogen and progesterone continue but there is no shedding. The menstruation stops and a woman is said to have conceived. The fertilized ovum gradually grows into the fetus and it takes about 266 days for a fertilized egg to grow into a baby. There are various types of deliveries.

Normal vaginal delivery

It is aided with a small cut of the vaginal outlet sometimes, the process in known as Episiotomy, which is done to help quicker delivery and undue downward pressure on uterus and adjoining parts like bladder and rectum. A normal delivery is generally done with a small cut at the vaginal outlet.

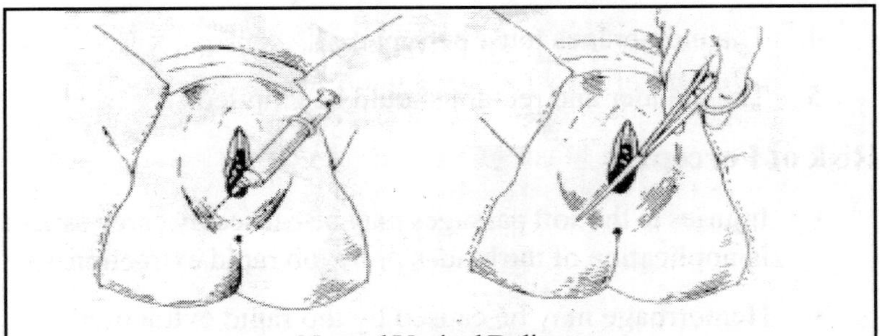

Normal Vaginal Delivery

Suction delivery

It is a process in which suction is applied to the low descending head of the baby to hasten deliver. It is also called vacuum method of delivery and helps the mother to deliver quickly. Anesthesia is not required in most of the cases.

Forceps delivery

In which baby's head is helped out with the use of forceps e.g. a large pair of tongs, which grasp the baby's head for applying a downward pull. Mild anesthesia is given to the mother to avoid excessive pain. The following are essential conditions for the application of Forceps:

1. The cervix must be fully dilated.
2. The head should be in the cavity of pelvis.
3. The head should be in a suitable position. A forceps delivery must not be attempted until the

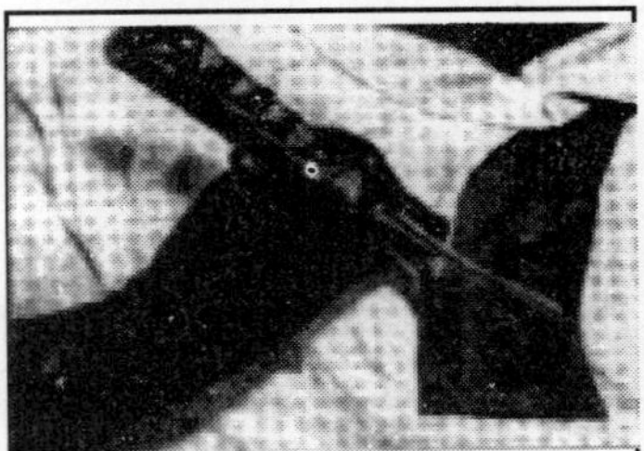

Forceps Delivery

operator is quite certain of the presentation and position of the head.

4. The membranes must be ruptured.

5. The bladder and rectum should be emptied.

Risk of Forceps:

- Injuries to the soft passages may be caused by carelessness in application of the blades or by too rapid extraction.
- Hemorrhage may be caused by too rapid extraction.
- Injuries to the child (e.g. fractures of the skull, intra-cranial hemorrhage, injury to eyes, facial paralysis, sphyxia for compression of head).

Multiple pregnancy

Do you have any history of multiple births in the family? If yes, then you must watch out and tell your doctor to diagnose seriously. It can be diagnosed by the size of womb or pelvic examination or USC scanning of abdomen. In case of signs of a multiple pregnancy, visit your doctor more frequently and have complete rest between 30th to 37th weeks, to avoid premature delivery. A multiple pregnancy means an extra trouble and sometimes there is a possibility of a caesarean section. Plural births require highly skilled pediatric care. The fetal mortality is much higher; pre-maturity, pro-lapse of the cord and asphyxia of the second twin takes a high toll. Congenital abnormalities in uniovular twins are common. Locked Twins is a rare complication, where the first child presents by the breech and the second by the head.

Delivery of the head

This is the critical phase, because delay may cause havoc. The reasons for the delay are the following:

- The head passes into the pelvic cavity, it is no longer subject to the expulsive power of the uterus.

- That the passage of head is resisted by the ring of vulva outlet. To avoid such risk, episiotomy should always be made in a primigravida when the buttocks are distending the perineum. However, when the child is small and the maternal passages roomy, spontaneous delivery may occur without giving a cut at the outlet of vagina.

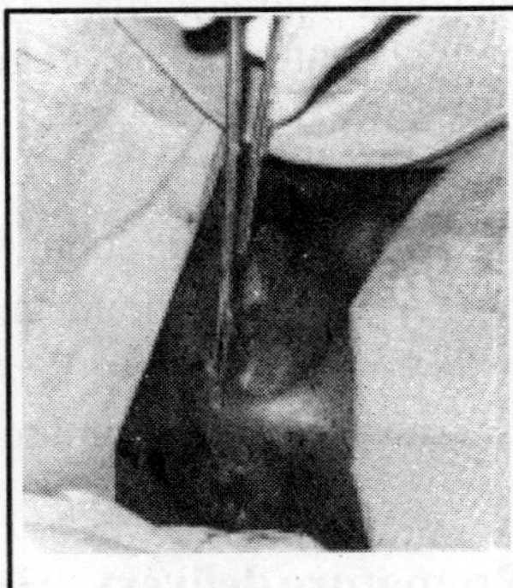
Epiciotomy

The usual method of delivery is to hold the child's body slightly downwards, straddled over the left hand and forearm, and exert gentle supra-pubic pressure on the head as the head enters the pelvic cavity. Gentle traction will deliver the face and head.

Ectopic or tubal delivery

It is a rare complication in which the fertilized ovum or embryo becomes blocked in its passage through the fallopian tube. There the embryo continues to grow as it normally would within the uterus. However, the space between the tubes is too small to allow expansion that may rupture, causing a serious hemorrhage and also intense pain in the pelvis. This may also result acute appendicitis. Consult a doctor for necessary surgery as soon as a tubal pregnancy is suspected before the occurrence of hemorrhage. Ectopic pregnancy remains one of the leading causes of maternal death, the classical triad of pain, abnormal vaginal

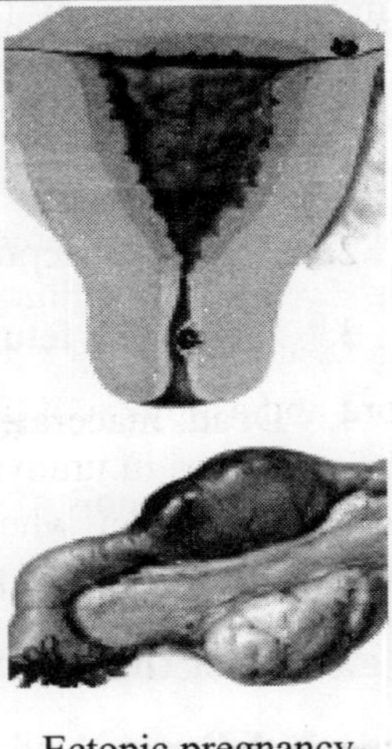
Ectopic pregnancy

bleeding and a palpable adnexal mass is present in most of the patients with ectopic pregnancy.

Induced delivery

In this connection, labor is brought on or induced artificially by rupturing the membranes and letting out a little amniotic fluid, which stimulates labor pains. When the pains are too feeble or the delivery is overdue, labor is induced by administrating medicines, which contract the uterus.

Premature delivery

The termination of pregnancy after the fetus has become viable such as capable to live independently, is called premature birth. And if the fetus is born dead, it is still-birth. Causes which produce abortions can endanger the growth of the fetus resulting in still birth or a premature delivery. Premature delivery is usually the problem with the placenta to the faulty blood supply to the fetus, defective hormone production and effect of injurious toxins and chemicals through the blood to the fetus. The causes of premature delivery are the following:

1. Obliquity of the uterus.
2. Uterus subseptus.
3. Premature fetus.
4. Dead, macerated and flaccid fetus.
5. Hydramnois
6. Placenta praevia.
7. Pelvic Tumor.

Breech delivery

Most babies are born in head-first position instead of feet-first or shoulder first. If the birth canal is adequate and the baby is small, there may not be any serious difficulty because of breech position. If the unborn baby is bulky and the birth outlet is small, this could be dangerous to both mother and the baby. Avoid traveling or bulky jerks during the last few days.

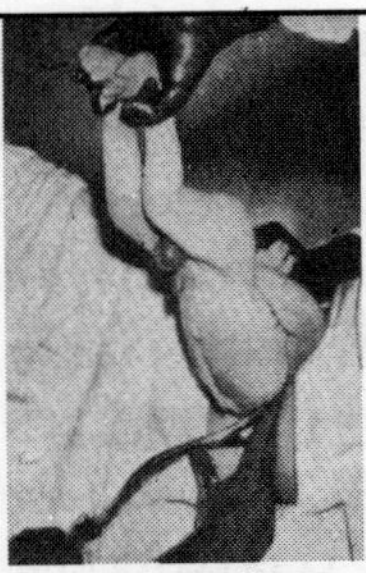

Breech Delivery

Internal version

1. Membrane intact or not ruptured recently. Avoid internal version in such cases.
2. The abdominal and uterine walls must be relaxed.
3. An anesthesia should always be given.
4. The cervix must be dilated sufficiently to admit the entire hand in uterus.
5. The position of the fetus must have been exactly mapped out by the palpation before the hand is introduced in the uterus.
6. The vulva and the vagina must be thoroughly cleansed.
7. Sterile rubber gloves should be worn.

Pass the hand into the uterus in cone-shape and seize a foot. The patient should be placed on her side or her back. If the knee is felt, the foot or knee should be brought down through the cervix. The head must be pushed up into the fundus of uterus by external hand.

Vaginal hysterotomy

This process is artificial dilation of the cervix is conducted by the fingers or by hydrostatic bags in the first stage is an operation, which has been nowadays been almost replaced by caesarean section - better and a safer operation.

Under general anesthesia the cervix is exposed by adequate vaginal retraction. With the scissors the cervix is cut at points in clockwise direction. The cut extends to the junction of the cervix and the vaginal wall. Following delivery by the forceps the cut is carefully sutured. The final results of the healing are usually unsatisfactory and lead to reverse hemorrhage sometimes. Incision of the cervix is now very uncommon operation. Attempt to dilate the cervix by the fingers is always almost followed by cervical lacerations and the operation of the incision of the cervix is always to be preferred.

How to do vaginal hysterotomy?

This operation has been almost entirely supplemented by abdominal hysterotomy. The steps of the operation are sufficiently indicated by the illustration here as described below:

1. Cervix drawn forcibly down longitudinal and transverse incisions in anterior vaginal wall.
2. Dissection of bladder from uterus and vaginal wall.
3. Splitting cervix anteriorly in which bladder and vaginal wall drawn up by the anterior retractor.
4. Cervix split anteriorly when the membranes bulge down.
5. Posterior incision sutured.

Displacement of uterus

It may be diagnosed by:

- Increase in backward displacement.
- Pain on micturition occurs, passing into retention if incarceration occurs.
- Undue enlargement of abdomen.

Generally, the enlargement of uterus and abdomen occurs due to pregnancy plus large tumor, hydramnnios, multiple pregnancy or even a mere mistake as to the date of conception. The bladder must be carefully emptied by catheter before examination.

How to treat displacement and abnormalities of uterus?

1. If by 12th week the uterus is still retroverted, then a large ring pessary is inserted into the vagina.
2. The patient is instructed to adopt the semi-prone position and remain in bed for a couple of days in the Sim's Position. It is found after 24 to 48 hours the fundus can be felt in the abdomen. The pessary should be left in vagina until after the 16th week of pregnancy (under doctor's supervision).

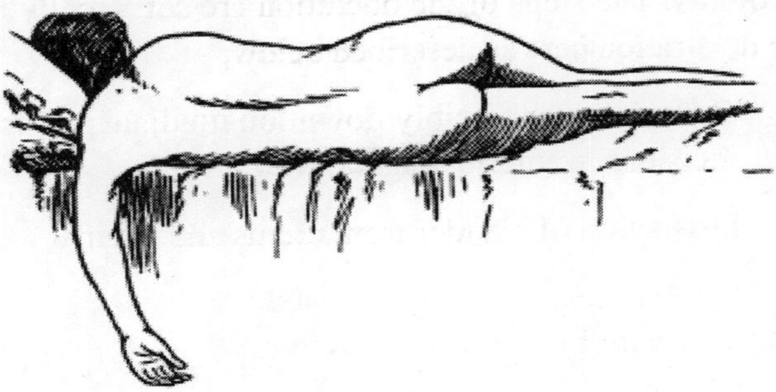

The Sim's Position

3. If the uterus remains retroverted after 48 hours, then manual reposition of the uterus may be undertaken. Simple manual reposition is done by inserting two fingers in the posterior fornix and pushing the fundus upwards and forwards. The cervix is then caught backwards by one finger and the other hand on the abdomen to catch the fundus. After the uterus has been replaced a large ring pessary should be inserted and not removed until after the 16th week of pregnancy.

4. In case of patient with a history of previous abortions, a laparotomy should be done immediately.

Abnormalities of uterus

The malformations of the uterus are usually the result of incomplete fusion of two mullerian ducts or of incomplete absorption of the septum between them. The complications recorded include a high incidence of abortion and premature labor, of inertia during labor, retained placenta, of transverse lies and breech presentations. There are several types of major developmental abnormalities of the uterus.

7

Physical Examination During Pregnancy

The doctor often asks certain questions regarding the previous pregnancy such as difficulty in previous delivery, abortions or miscarriages (if any) in past, the birth of premature or macerated fetuses or death of children occurring in early infancy (if an), the blood of both parents should be examined and the [patient should be questioned about her present health, existence of cardiac or pulmonary disease or toxaemia, for example breathlessness, palpitation, cough, excessive vomiting, persistent headaches, swelling of the hands or face, diminished amount of urine, dimness of vision, condition of the bowels, the presence of vaginal discharges and their nature, swelling of the feet or legs, presence of hemorrhoids or varicose veins etc. should be enquired into.

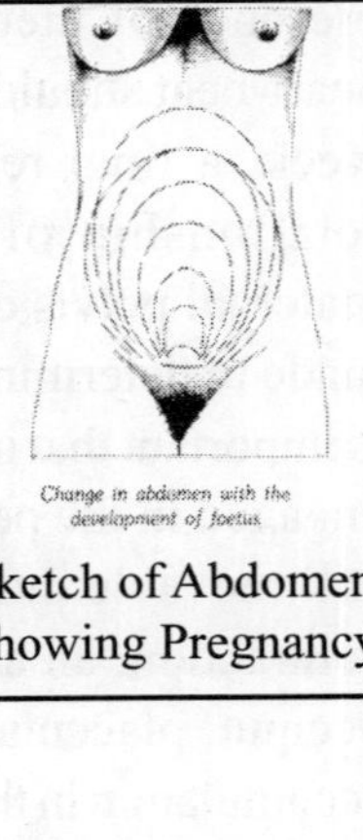
Change in abdomen with the development of foetus

Sketch of Abdomen Showing Pregnancy

After preliminary questioning is finished, the patient is asked to undress and lie upon an examination couch. Firstly, a general survey of circulatory, respiratory and digestive system is made. See that the doctor inspects the breast noting their development, the condition of nipples, areola (the darkish part around nipples) and the presence and the amount of secretion from them (if any). The mouth should always be examined for septic teeth, gums and tonsils. The blood pressure should then be estimated frequently. It is important to find out blood group of the expectant mother for investigation of hemoglobin and Rh group.

The patient's height is recorded and it may be worthwhile to mention that women of short stature (five feet or below) are more likely to have small pelvis than taller women. The patient's weight is noted and a check on weight gain is made during the pregnancy.

Abdominal examination

In early pregnancy, note the size of uterus and exclude any morbid abdominal conditions. Prior to the 26th week of pregnancy abdominal diagnosis of presentation and position is often inaccurate. The level of the fundus, the presence of uterine soufflé, hearing the heart-beat should be examined. At the 38th week, a final review is carried out and relationship of the fetal head to the maternal pelvis determined. A study is be made to determine the size of the head related to the pelvis brim. It is important that in a primigravida, the head should normally become engaged in the pelvis during the last two or three weeks. It may be still movable during the last fortnight of pregnancy due to pelvic contraction, an abnormally large head, a posterior position of the occiput, placenta praevia, a pelvic tumor or simply due to faecal accumulation in the pelvic colon and rectum. A thorough examination of abdominal region should be conducted by the doctor to find out if the head is able to enter the pelvis.

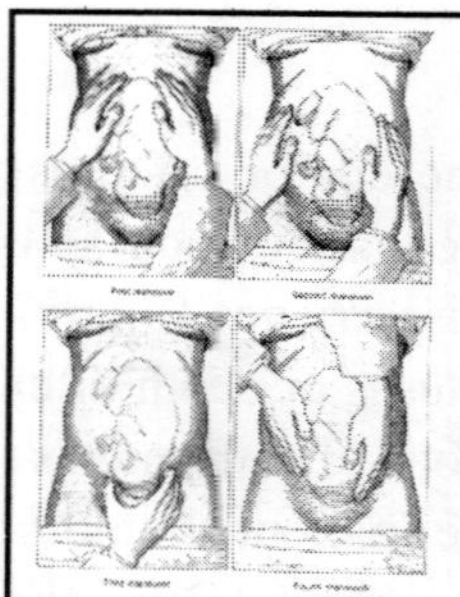

4 Positions of Abdomen

Pelvic examination

The objects are twofold- to investigate the condition of the pelvic organs and to estimate the size and shape of the pelvic canal. It is necessary to measure the pelvis by your doctor by means of a bimanual examination. The diagnosis of pregnancy is confirmed and the presence or absence of pelvic swellings such as uterine fibroids or ovarian cysts can be determined. If the fundus of the uterus can be palpated abdominally there is no need to carry out the pelvic examination at the first visit and can be postponed until need arises. There are three methods of pelvic examination as below:

1. **External examination:** The measurements are made with a pair of calipers to find out any deformity to be recognized at once.
2. **Internal examination**: Interspinous diameter is measured with calipers. The two, anterior-superior spines are located, where the points of caliper are placed on their outer lips and the measurement read off. Normally it is 9-1/2 to 10 inches (24 –25 cm.). The Intercristal diameter is also measured at the points passed slowly round the iliac cresta until the points of greatest separation are found when the measurement is read normally, it is 10-1/2 to 11 inches (26-27 cm.).
3. **By X-rays**: The size of the pelvis and the fetal head can be assessed by X-ray. This process is known as Radiographic Pelvimetry.

Blood pressure

The blood pressure of the patient should be ascertained at each antenatal visit. During pregnancy the blood pressure should not rise above 140/90. If after a suitable period of rest, the pressure remains above this figure, then hypertension is said to exist. During the middle trimester of pregnancy the blood pressure is often low and the reading of 11o/70 may be recorded. This physiological drop is of great interest and is called the 'mid pregnancy drop' in blood pressure.

Urine and hemoglobin

Usually, the patient is asked to pass water before she undresses for the physical examination. Examination of urine is most important throughout pregnancy. The possible presence of albumin is most important point to attend to, besides checking the presence of sugar, pus and other abnormalities. Urine should be examined once a month in the first six months, thereafter more frequently as pregnancy advances. If the albumin is present in the urines along with a vaginal discharge, a mid-stream specimen of urine should be obtained and a doctor should be consulted. The hemoglobin should be checked throughout pregnancy. It should be estimated as routine in all pregnant women at the 30th week. If you are suffering from anemia, there is plenty of time to correct this. All Rh Negative patients have their blood examined for the presence of antibodies at regular intervals.

Weight

Be carefully when the weight increases during pregnancy, since fluid retention in the tissues along with the increase in weight, is the earliest signs of toxaemia. In normal pregnancy, the increase in weight begins with the 4th month and continues at an average rate of about 2 kg per month to about the 39th week, the total weight being about 12 kg. Any abnormal gain in weight should determine a careful investigation.

Vaginal secretion

The vaginal secretion in a healthy pregnancy differs only in its increased quantity from that of a healthy non-pregnant woman. It is whitish in color, containing epithelial cells, leucocytes and mucus. It also contains numerous large 'vaginal bacilli'. It has been observed that the acidity of the vaginal secretion is inimical to the life of other organism than the 'vaginal bacillus', followed by the appearance of organism in the vagina. Thus during the puerperium the lochia (discharge from the uterus after labor) is alkaline, which contain many organisms, mostly saprophytic are found.

Method of cleaning genitals

The birth canal can be divided into three parts:

1. The vulva which may be designated the septic tract.
2. The vaginal area has acidic secretions, fungi and leucocytes. This is also Antiseptic Tract.
3. The cavity of the uterus, separated by the plug of mucus from the vagina, is entirely devoid of any form of organism. It is therefore the Aseptic Tract.

Cleansing of vulva

Wherever possible the patient should have a complete bath at the very commencement of labor, and the nurse should see that the rectum and bladder are emptied. It is usually suggested that the patient should be given an enema in every case, irrespective of whether the bowels have acted naturally or not, unless the patient is in strong labor when the nurse arrives. The nurse should then pay special attention to the genitals. The hair should be shaved. Before a vaginal examination is made the vulva is swabbed with a antiseptic solution. The labia minora must be separated and wiped with pledgets of wool soaked in an antiseptic solution always be drawn from being backwards to prevent carrying forward any septic matter from near the anus. No pledget must be used for more than one wipe.

Puerperal infection

The term puerperal infection can be used to describe any infection during or after labor, it generally applies to infection of the uterus and surrounding tissues after delivery. This can vary from mild to life threatening in severity. Some of the most severe infections may appear within hours of the delivery and are often opportunistic and non-associated with reliable risk factors. Vigilance and aggressive diagnosis and treatment are required. The puerperal infection causes due to colonization and infection of the tissues of uterus, peritoneum or surrounding organs. Abscesses usually contain both aerobic and anaerobic bacteria. Nearly 50% of the ascending uterine infections involve Chlamydia trachomatis. The risk factors of this infection includes a Cesarean delivery, invasive procedure during labor, prolonged rupture of the membranes, prolonged labor, multiple examinations, retained placental fragments, urinary catheter, intravenous line, low socioeconomic status and chronic diseases including diabetes.

The signs and symptoms of the infection are fever and tachycardia often developing rapidly after delivery, uterine tenderness, sign of septic or cardiovascular shock, hypertension, anxiety, disorientation, prostration, impaired renal function, hemolysis or hemoconcentration. The infection can be diagnosed by the following:

1. Urinary tract infection, including Pyelonephritis, in which large numbers of white blood cells and cultures are positive.
2. Wound infection.
3. Infection in intravenous line or site, contaminated fluids.
4. Disturbed abscess.
5. Septic thrombophlebitis.
6. Necrotizing fascitis.
7. Transfusion reaction.
8. Amniotic fluid or pulmonary embolism.
9. Cardiogenic shock.
10. Toxic shock syndrome.
11. Mastitis.
12. Afelectasis.

Possible associated conditions include septic shock, adult respiratory distress syndrome, acute renal failure and disseminated intra-vascular coagulation.

Vaginal examination

The use of abdominal palpation instead of this method of examination in normal cases has already been recommended. Where a vaginal examination is necessary it must be done with care. The patient should be on her back rather than on her side, so as to diminish the risk of the hand coming into contact with the anus. Cleanse hands and vulva before conducting the examination. The labia minora is separated apart by the left hand fingers. The fingers of right hand are introduced in the vagina without coming into contact with vulva at all, or at least only the inner surfaces of the labia minora, which have also been cleansed. In case, the patient is passing through the stage of labor, it is well to introduce the fingers into the vagina during a pain and prolong the examination until it passes off. One can learn the state of matters both during and between pains. Ascertain the following points during vaginal examination:

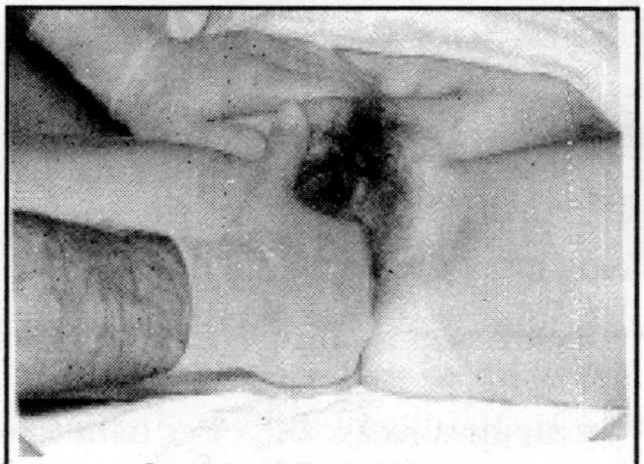

Bimanual Examination

1. State of labor; how far advanced it is?
2. Presentation and position?
3. Are the membranes ruptured? (in case not, be careful not to rupture the same).
4. State of vagina and perineum to check rigidity, moistness or dryness.
5. Is pelvis normal?
6. Is cord prolapsed?

8

40 Weeks of Pregnancy

How pregnancy develops?

The upper broad end of the uterus opens on either side into two long tubes called the fallopian tubes, each ending in a funnel shaped opening guarded by five finger-like projections called fibria, which lies close to the ovary - a spherical walnut sized organ producing female hormones and eggs called ova. Ovulation occurs usually in the middle of a menstrual cycle (middle between two consecutive periods). At birth, each ovary has thousands of follicles and each follicle is capable of giving one mature egg. During a woman's reproductive life about 400 ova are shed. When ovulation occurs, the ovum is picked up and travels down the fallopian tube towards the uterine cavity.

Menstruation is a process of 28-day cycle in which follicle matures and ovaries produce oestrogenic hormones. When an ovum matures, it is shed and starts traveling. The follicle, which contains this ovum produce the hormone progesterone. In case there is no pregnancy, the level of the hormones falls and is shed off along with the blood. This is called menstruation.

Fertilization is the union of a mature ovum with sperm. If sexual intercourse takes place within 12 to 24 hours of ovulation, then one of the thousands of sperms deposited in vagina unites with the ovum to fertilize it after traveling down uterine cavity and reaching the fallopian tube. Once the pregnancy has got established, the production of hormones: estrogen and progesterone continues but there is no shedding. The menstruation stops and a woman is said to have conceived.

Enhancing sex power through therapeutic baths

Type of bath	Water temperature	Genital advantages
Cold Hip Bath	10-18 degree C	Cures irregular menstruation, uterine infection, pelvic inflammation, prostate glands, seminal weakness in men, impotency, sterility, ovary and uterine displacement.
Hot Hip Bath	40-50 degree C	Cures pelvic inflammation, chronic urine infection, irregularities of menstruation, impotency in men, disorders of ovaries and uterus.
Epsom salt bath	1.5 kg salt in water	Cures genital diseases and kidney disorders.
Alternate Hip Bath	hot followed by cold	Chronic inflammation in the pelvic viscera, ovaries, genito-urinary organs and cellulite.
Neutral Hip Bath	30-36 degree C	Inflammations of bladder, urethra, uterus, ovaries, fallopian tubes, testicles, painful spasms of the vagina and pruritis of the anus and vulva.
Mud bath		Cure venereal diseases.

Three stages of pregnancy

The delivery dater is generally 280 days after the first day of the last period. The 40- week period of pregnancy is classified into three trimesters as below:

- The first trimester: Period starting from 1st to 12th week.
- The second trimester starts from 13th week to 28th week.
- The third trimester starting from 29th to 40th week

The child in womb becomes theoretically capable of living a separate individual existence about the 28th week of pregnancy. It is important to know the age of a fetus or embryo both for clinical and medico reasons.

- At the end of 4th week: The embryo is much curved, head and tail being close together. It measures from 2.5 to 4 mm. from crown to rump. The brain and the cord are enclosed, eye and ear vesicles are visible. The heart is prominent and is beginning to divide in four chambers.
- At t the end of 8th week: The embryo is about an inch (25 mm.) long in crown rump measurement. The head has a human shape, whereas the tail has nearly disappeared. The hands and feet begin to appear. Eyes, nose and ears are recognizable. The external genitals are visible, but sex is not distinguishable. The embryo now becomes the fetus.
- At the end of 12th week: The fetus is about 3-1/2 to 4 inches long weighing about 50 gm. The intestines are enclosed in the abdomen and umbilical cord is beginning to show spiral turns. Sex can be determined by the presence or absence of the uterus. Most of the bones are beginning to show centers of ossification.
- At the end of 16th week: The fetus is about six inches (15 cm.) long and weighs about 190 gm. Sex is clearly defined at this stage. The fine downy hair starts appearing on the

skin.

- At the end of20th week: The fetus is about 7 to 8 inches (18-20 cm.) long weighing about 450 gm. The head is still relatively large. The cord is about 12 inches long.
- At the end of 24th week: The fetus is about 9 inches (23 cm.) long and weighs about 930 gm. Fat begins to deposit under the skin. Hair appears on the head.
- At the end of 28th week: The fetus is about eleven inches (28 cm.) long weighing about 1300 gm. The eyelids are now open and the papillary membrane starts disappearing. The body is now covered with fine hair (lanugo). The intestines contain a dark green tarry matter known as meconium. A child born at this time very seldom survives.
- At the end of 32nd week: The fetus is nearly 12 inches long weighing about 2075 gm. The hair on the scalp is thicker.
- At the end of 36th week: The length of fetus is nearly 14 inches weighing about 2500 gm. The subcutaneous fat has increased, and the face is less wrinkled and the body more round. A child born at this time has a very fair chance of survival.
- At the 40th week: The total length reaches 20 inches weighing about 3200 gm. The fingers have complete nail, the skin is pink and smooth. The diameter of the head becomes normal. In the male the testicles are in the scrotum.

Prenatal examinations

The following tests and examinations are performed at the first or second prenatal visit to doctor, which helps assure the birth of healthy baby:

- complete medical history and physical examination.
- A pelvic (vaginal) examination to confirm pregnancy,

estimate the size and shape of your pelvis, to do a Pap smear to detect cervical cancer and to test for gonorrhea.

- Blood test to determine your blood type, Rh factor, test for anemia, infection, syphilis and German measles immunity.
- Urine test to check protein, sugar and any infection.
- At each prenatal monthly visit to your doctor check up for weight, blood pressure, urine and abdominal examination to measure the growth of uterus, fetus and estimate the size and position of fetus should be carried out.

Warning signs during pregnancy

Warning signs	Possible problems
* Vaginal bleeding	Miscarriage, placenta previa, abruption placenta and premature labor.
* Abdominal pain	Ectopic pregnancy, abruption placentae and premature labor contractions.
* Leakage of fluid from vagina	Rupture of membranes.
* Sudden puffiness or body swelling	Pre-eclampsia (toxemia).
* Severe, persistent headache	Pre-eclampsia (toxemia)
* Disturbance of vision, spots And flashes	Pre-eclampsia (toxemia)
* Dizziness	Pre-eclampsia or supine hypo-tension.
* Pain or burning on urination	Urinary tract infection and sexually transmitted disease (STD).

* Vaginal discharge, sores or itching	Vaginal infection and STD.
* Fever (oral temperature)	Infection.
* Persistent nausea	Hyperemesis gravidarum and infection.
* Reduction in fetal activity	Fetal distress.

First trimester of pregnancy

The important sign and symptoms include:

- Missed period, but sometimes the pregnant woman keeps having their periods two to three months after they conceive.
- Nausea and vomiting, many times, such women do not have nausea and vomiting.
- Exhaustion, tiredness and excessive giddiness all the time.
- Morning sickness.
- Change of taste.
- Strong liking and disliking for certain foods.
- Frequent urge to urinate.
- Engorged and tender breasts.
- Increase of discharge from nipples.

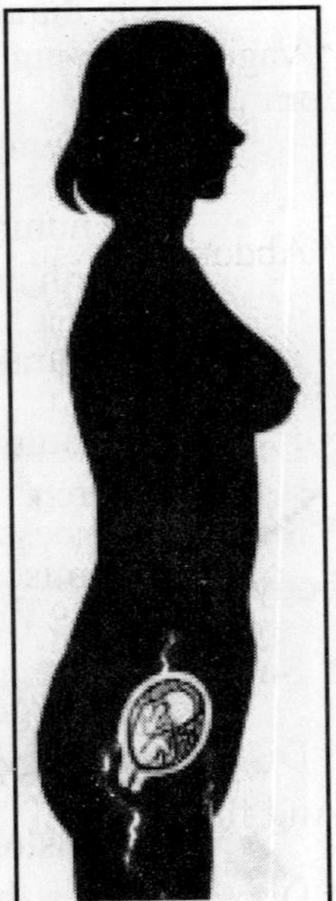

First Trimester

After conceiving, the fertilized egg travels down the fallopian tube to get embedded in the lining of the womb in the 3rd week. By the 6th week, the embryo is 1.25 cm long but doesn't look like a baby. It has large head with pits for eyes and a tail. By the 12th week the baby measures about

9 cm weighing approximately 9 gm. It appears like a human embryo with all internal organs. The fetus takes nutrition from the mother and discharges its waste material into her blood through placenta. Always take medicines as prescribed by a doctor. Placenta, full of blood vessels, is formed partly by the fetal and partly by the uterine tissues. Placenta also produces hormones necessary for the substance of pregnancy. After baby's birth the placenta gets separated from the uterine wall and is expelled from the uterus.

On finding the symptoms of pregnancy, the pregnant woman should consult a doctor and tell him/her the following:

- The date of the first day of last menstruation period.
- The duration and heaviness in menstrual flow having in past.
- Any complication faced in previous pregnancies.
- The number of children and their usual weight at the time of birth in previous cases of pregnancy.
- The duration of lactation (breast feeding) in past cases.
- The number of years of marriage and the number of children.
- Any miscarriage or termination of pregnancy too place in past.
- If undergoing any treatment at the present or in past. In case of a past surgery, inform the doctor.
- Past history of health with detail of prolonged suffering such as diabetes, high blood pressure, epilepsy or heart disease.
- If you or your husband or any close blood relation is suffering from a hereditary or venereal disease.
- If ever exposed to X-rays.

- If you are anemic.
- If suffering from cystitis (painful and embarrassing condition in which there is a frequent urge to urinate.
- Any abnormal condition such as frequent pain an abdomen or pelvic region, blood discharge, white discharge accompanied with mucus. Boils or itching around urinary opening, pain during intercourse, irregular menses or any other condition.

A pregnant woman must undergo the following monthly tests/ examination by the doctor:

- Weight gain.
- Recording blood pressure.
- Oral hygiene checked regularly.
- Signs of anemia, swelling of legs, feet and hands.
- Inspection of heart and lungs.
- Examination of breasts to check for any lumps and abnormality of nipples.
- Vaginal examination. During the first 12 weeks the uterus cannot be felt by placing hand on abdomen. To confirm pregnancy, an internal pelvic examination has to be performed between 6th and 10th week of pregnancy.

To find correct picture and determine the size of the uterus gently inserting two gloved fingers into the vagina and pushing firmly on abdomen to assess the uterus thoroughly. The patient is made to lie flat on the examination table bending legs in such a way so as to keep the feet on the table and pelvic muscles relaxed.

A pregnant woman should avoid the following during first trimester:

- Wearing tight clothes.

- Drinking excessive tea and coffee.
- Jerky or long traveling.
- Over-exertion.
- X-rays.
- Strong medicines without doctor's prescription.
- Smoking or drinking.
- Standing for a long time or getting up suddenly from sitting position.
- Contact with animals, especially cats and birds, which may lead to abortion, premature delivery or birth of a sickly baby.
- Not consulting the doctor on finding symptoms such as bleeding or excessive discharge through vagina, abdominal pain, painful burning urination, persistent vomiting, frequent fever and feeling of dizziness. If you feel dizzy sit down with your head between your toes.

A pregnant should take the following precautions during first trimester:

- A monthly check up and consultation with the doctor.
- Have frequent small meals – about 6 to 7 times a day.
- Get 8 to 10 hours sleep during night and minimum to hours rest during the day.
- Restrict fluid intake in the evening to avoid frequent urination during night.
- Hormonal changes lead to a feeling of lethargy and exhaustion during the first trimester of pregnancy, so a complete rest is essential in this period.
- Consult a doctor in case of burning sensation while passing

urine.

- Eat hygienically cooked food.
- Relax for few minutes with your feet up during lunch hours.
- Take anti-vomiting drug in consultation with the doctor in case of severe nausea and vomiting.

How to do a vaginal examination?

Where a vaginal examination is necessary it must be done with care. The patient should be on her back rather than on her side, so as to diminish the risk of the hand coming into contact with the anus. Cleanse hands and vulva before conducting the examination. The labia minora is separated apart by the left hand fingers. The fingers of right hand are introduced in the vagina without coming into contact with vulva at all, or at least only the inner surfaces of the labia minora, which also need cleansing.

Second trimester of pregnancy

Signs and symptoms during 2nd trimester include the following:

- No nausea and vomiting.
- Desire to urinate frequently subsides.
- Movement of growing baby in the womb is noticed by the 18th week in case of first delivery, otherwise by the 16th week of pregnancy.
- Enlargement of breasts visible.

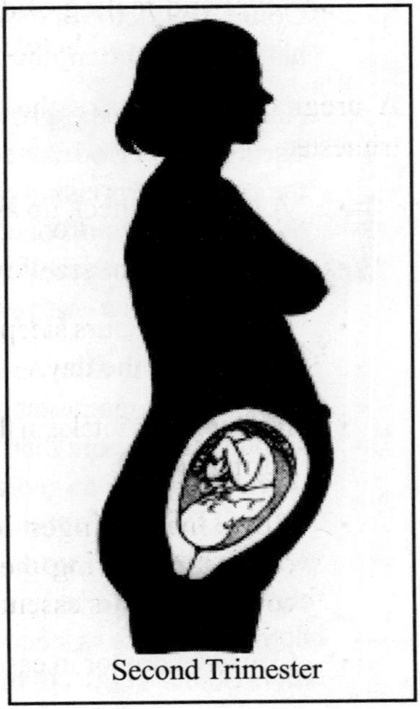

Second Trimester

- Gradual increase of bulge in abdomen.
- Skin around the nipples becomes dark.
- Clear watery secretion from nipples becomes thick and yellowish when squeezing by the 16th week.
- Small, pinkish and white streaks become visible on the lower abdomen.
- The skin of the upper thighs gets stretched by the 20th week.
- Appetite lost during 1st trimester of pregnancy returns. There is 20-25% increase in appetite of a pregnant woman during the last trimester of pregnancy.

Some essential checks during 2nd trimester of pregnancy are the following:

- Have a regular check over the blood pressure as during pregnancy it is slightly lower than pre-pregnancy stage. Consult a doctor in case blood pressure start rising as it is harmful for the mother as well as the baby.
- A check over the growth of baby in womb is essential during this period. After 12th week the womb lying deep in the pelvis starts rising out of bony pelvis, which can be felt by placing a hand on the lower abdomen. A doctor may easily assess the size of womb and the baby besides having a check if it is a multiple pregnancy.
- Check weight after the first trimester of pregnancy. The total weight gain during three trimesters of pregnancy should not be more than 10 to 12 kg. After the first trimester, there should be an increase in weight ranging from 0.7 to 1.4 kg. On completion of 20 weeks, the total increase in weight should be up to 4 kg. In case of lesser weight than the normal required gain, it indicates poor growth of the baby and there is need for the improvement in mother's diet. If the weight is more than the normal gain coupled

with increase in blood pressure, consult a doctor immediately. Avoid excessive intake of wrong kind of food.

- Ensure regular urine test for proteins as you may be suffering from pre-eclamptic toxaemia (PET), which is common disorder in expectant mothers having high blood pressure.
- Around the 7th week of pregnancy visit your doctor for an ultrasound. You can hear baby's heartbeats around the 14th week of pregnancy. The doctor must observe the rate and rhythm of the baby's heartbeats.
- Urine test is a must to find out the traces of sugar every month, indicating diabetes and functioning of kidneys.
- Swelling of hands, ankles and legs should be examined by your doctor every time you go for check up once a month. Have a hemoglobin test to detect early signs of anemia, if any and should be treated accordingly.
- Even in case of a normal pregnancy, between 16th to 20th week of pregnancy, a routine ultrasound scan is advised to find out the growth of the child and position of placenta. In case the position of placenta is near or on the cervical opening there are chances of severe bleeding and immediate attention of a doctor is required.
- Carry out alpha feto protein test during 15th to 18th week of pregnancy. Alpha feto protein is a substance produced by the baby, which passes into the mother's blood stream. There are chances of congenital defect or there may be two babies in the womb, in case of abnormally high levels of this protein.
- Amniocentosis test is carried out between the 14th to 18th week of pregnancy to detect any abnormality in the baby. It is carried out only when the age of the expectant mother is more than 35 years and has delivered a malformed baby previously.

- During 2nd trimester of pregnancy, tetanus toxoid injections are administered twice at an interval of one month.

Avoid the following during 2nd trimester of pregnancy:

- Do not take greasy and spicy foods to avoid chances of excessive weight gain.
- Drink 7 to 8 glasses of water a day.
- Avoid constipation.
- Avoid excessive intake of sugar and salt.
- Avoid canned and processed foods. Take extra fruits and pulses.
- Avoid eating at unhygienic places.
- Sexual intercourse is not permissible in the 2nd trimester of pregnancy in case of previous miscarriage or in case of vaginal bleeding. However, normal sex is permissible within the physical constraints imposed by the growing womb. A pregnant woman can, however, fulfill her husband's needs with love and tenderness, omitting intercourse.
- Avoid strenuous exercises in this trimester. Start with light exercises for 5 minutes and gradually increase the duration to 20 minutes.
- Take complete bed rest if bleeding occurs.
- Do not exert to the point where you get tired. A walk in the open in the early morning is the best exercise during this trimester. Besides the physical toning up, it has a calming and relaxing effect.
- Do not wear high-heeled shoes. Wear flat shoes as far as possible.
- Do not bend your waist while picking up any object from the ground. Keep your back straight and bend at your knees and hips.

3rd trimester of pregnancy

The period from 29th to 40th week of pregnancy is the last stage and need a lot of care. As the arrival of new baby draws nearer, expecting mothers are filled with excitement to see the new arrival as well as the fear of the delivery of child. The expectant mother should visit a doctor once a week in case of any complication or once in a fortnight in case of normal condition. During the final month of pregnancy between 37th to 40th weeks, the following medical check up and precautions are essential:

- There must be three or more movements of the baby in one hour during the last week of pregnancy. In case the movements are less, consult your doctor.
- Get checked blood pressure and urine.
- Check any swelling on the face and feet and inform your doctor.
- Consult your doctor for finding the position of the baby in the womb, size and growth, heartbeats of the baby etc. by an abdominal examination. These information help during the process of delivery.
- In case you find any abnormality in breast nipples, consult your

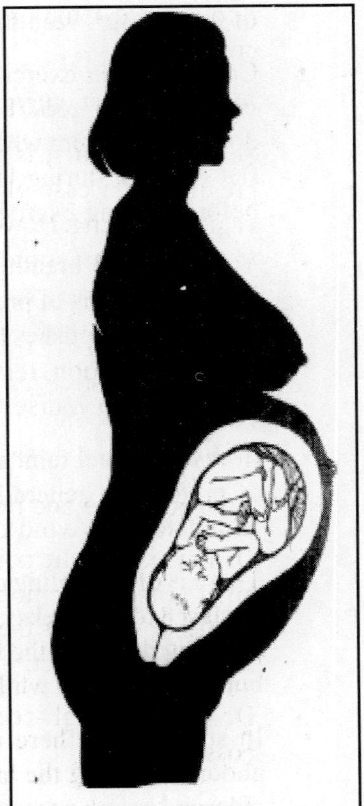

Third Trimester

doctor. A nipple exercise will be beneficial to treat disorder.

- Avoid sex during this period as it becomes cumbersome and physically difficult because of bulging abdomen. Sex should strictly be avoided if there is a history of bleeding during pregnancy or there is risk of premature birth of baby or such a thing has happened in the past. However, there is no harm if the intercourse is done carefully after consulting your doctor, lying in such a position that there is no pressure on the abdomen, preferably in a position having back to your partner.
- Take 8 to 10 hours of sleep during the night and minimum of 3 to 4 hours rest during the day.
- Continue light exercises during this trimester, which are important for good health. Make sure the exercises are done to the extent where you do not get tired. Avoid lying flat on back during late pregnancy. Consult your doctor before starting exercise.
- You may feel breathlessness and discomfort during the last two months of pregnancy usually due to the growing womb, which pushes the other abdominal organs upward. In such condition, rest as much as possible. Use an extra pillow to prop yourself up while lying down.
- In case you feel faint and dizzy during the last four weeks of pregnancy generally due to low blood pressure, take complete rest. Avoid standing for a long period.
- There is often feeling of frequent urination during night in the last 8 to 10 weeks of pregnancy generally due to womb pressing down on the bladder. Do not worry if there is no burning sensation while passing urine.
- In some cases there is burning sensation in the upper abdomen during the last phase of pregnancy because the enlarged womb presses against the stomach, thus pushing food contents up into the food pipe resulting in pain and

burning sensation in the upper abdomen and below the ribs. To prevent this, avoid taking spicy and fried foods. Take smaller quantity of food at short intervals instead of taking heavy meals at long intervals.

- Leakage of urine on light jerk is another common problem during the last trimester of pregnancy due to weak pelvic floor below the womb. Avoid lifting heavy weights and constipation. Empty your bladder frequently. A light pelvic exercise will help a lot. To exercise pelvic, lie on the floor with back and knees bent so that your feet lie flat touching the floor. Now tighten the muscles by pressing hips and thighs drawing your vagina in as much as possible.
- Reddish, moist rashes may develop in the skin folds usually under the breasts and in the groin region) during the last stage of pregnancy (mostly in summer). The expectant mother should keep such area dry and clean and avoid use of nylon underwear. Always use cotton undergarments.
- Painful contraction of muscles, usually in the calves, is another problem during the last trimester of pregnancy generally due to deficiency of calcium. Take calcium tablets with the consultation of doctor. Massage the affected area and in case the calves are affected, walk for sometime to regulate blood circulation.
- Heavy swelling of the feet, fingers and other parts on the body usually occur in late pregnancy and is called pre-elcamptic toxemia (PET) – which is a combination of swelling on ankles, fingers and vulva (also known as oedema of vulva) followed by puffiness of the face with increased blood pressure and presence of protein in urine. The risk of PET is more common among obese women and females getting married in teenage. Women with family history of high blood pressure are prone to this risk and consult a doctor immediately. A delayed treatment may cause a risk of fits and birth of a retarded child.

- Expectant mother in the habit of smoking and drinking cause severe damage to the baby in the womb. Intra-uterine growth retardation is a condition where he growth of baby in womb is severely impaired due to anemia and malnourishment. To ensure a healthy baby, it is important to completely part with smoking and taking alcohol. Smoking is the root cause of certain diseases like high blood pressure, chronic kidney diseases, heart ailments and several infections harmful for mother as well as for the child's health and growth. Excessive smoking affects production of breast milk and alcohol taken by the mother passed into the baby causing severe side effects.

- The gums start bleeding and become inflamed during the last trimester of pregnancy. Brush your teeth thoroughly after taking meal and massage gums gently.

- There is a complaint of leakage of urine while walking briskly, laughing or sneezing by the expecting mothers during the last trimester of pregnancy due to loss of strength of muscles of the pelvic floor, which support the intestines, urinary bladder and womb. Here is an exercise to treat this disorder. Lie on the floor with back and knees bent keeping feet flat on the ground. Tighten the muscles, squeezing as if trying to stop the urine. Draw your vagina in, pause for a while and then relax. Repeat for 10 to 15 times.

- Expectant mothers develop the problem of piles in the last trimester of pregnancy due to constant pressure of the baby on blood vessels around anal region. This also results in soreness, itching pain and bleeding while passing stool. Avoid constipation and standing for a long time. Consult a doctor to prescribe an ointment to reduce pain and itching.

- The expectant mothers feel uneasy and cannot sleep properly in the night usually during the 3rd trimester of pregnancy. Reading or a warm bath before going to sleep helps a lot. Lie on your side with a pillow under the head.

- Constipation is another problem common during the 3rd trimester because the bowel movement slows down under the influence of progesterone hormone. As such the stools become hard and infrequent. Take plenty of fluids besides regular exercise. Avoid laxatives. Consult a doctor.

- Problem of excess sweating arise during the last trimester of pregnancy generally attributed to hormonal changes. Wear loose clothes, especially during night and take plenty of water.

- Many times, there is thick curd-like discharge with severe itching in the vaginal region. A slight increase in the clear or whitish vaginal secretion is normal. The hormonal changes during last trimester of pregnancy make one more prone to vaginal thrush with a thick discharge and itching, which make urination painful. Avoid use of soap and nylon undergarments and keep the area around the vagina dry.

- The risk of complications during delivery is more pronounced in women suffering from anemia. The red blood cells contain a substance called hemoglobin, which carries oxygen. The normal level of hemoglobin is 11 to 14 gm. In case its level falls to below 10 gm, one is considered anemic. An anemic expectant mother may have a smaller than the normal child or a premature baby. The risk of pregnancies also increases during delivery in anemic women.

- Multistage pregnancy can easily be diagnosed by the size of womb or USG scanning. In case of a multiple pregnancy consult your doctor more frequently and take complete rest between 30th to 37th weeks to avoid premature delivery. There may be a possibility of a caesarian section in case of a multiple pregnancy. In case of caesarian section the delivery of baby is made through an incision in the uterus rather than the baby's exit through cervix and vagina where incision is done in the low lying transverse region in the lower abdomen where the becomes hidden under pubic hair.

Pregnancy calendar at a glance

(First Trimester)

Fetal growth: After conception, up to four weeks the fetal length is about 1/4th inch. The eyes, ears, mouth, brain, spine, spinal cord and umbilical cord start forming. The heart starts beating by the 25th day. It is called **ovum** until two weeks. By the end of 8th week, the length of fetal grows up to 1-1/8 inches with the formation of arms, legs, bones, internal organs, the brain and tooth buds. It is called **embryo.** By the end of 12 weeks the fetal growth ranges to 3 inches long when the movement of arms and legs starts. The fingers and toes are formed. Can smile and frown, sex is distinguishable and can urinate. It is called a **fetus.**

Placental and uterine changes: Uterine lining becomes thick with increased blood supply. Uterus starts enlarging, cervix becomes softer, implantation of ovum is usually in upper back portion of uterus and there is formation of placenta and umbilical cord. By the end of 8 weeks, the uterus is of size of a tennis ball. By the end of 12 weeks the size of uterus is like a grapefruit, the fundus is just above pubic bone, amniotic fluids fills uterine cavity and is continually replaced. At this time there is complete exchange of nutrients and waste products through placenta. The placenta is the major source of estrogen and progesterone.

Common physical and emotional changes: The following changes are observed in expectant mother by the end of 12 weeks:

- No menstruation.
- Has fullness or ache in pelvis.
- May be nauseated and may vomit frequently.

- Feels tired.
- Has increased vaginal secretion.
- May feel faint.
- Urinate more frequently.
- Breasts are fuller, nipple may tingle and areola is darker.
- May lose or gain up to 2 to 2.5 kg.
- Moods widely vary.
- There is always focus on body changes
- Sexual relationship in both partners may change.
- May feel ambivalent towards pregnancy: joy and excitement vs. resentment and panic. Well-being of baby remains a concern in both partners.

(Second trimester)

Fetal growth: Till 16th week the fetal is 6 inches long with strong heart beats, active muscles, thin and transparent skin, downy hair covering the body, formation of fingernails and toenails. By the end of 20th week the fetal length reaches 10 to 12 inches and there is presence of hair, eyelashes and eyebrows. By the end of 24 week the fetal length reaches 11 to 14 inches, the skin gets wrinkled and the meconium starts collecting in bowel.

Placental and uterine changes: Till the end of 16th week the uterus is placed 3 inches above the pubic bone and the placenta performs nutritional, respiratory, excretory and most endocrine functions. The amniotic fluid increases in amount. By the end of 20th week, the uterus is placed at level of navel and the size of placenta covers half of the inner surface of uterus. By the end of 24 weeks the uterus reaches above the level of navel.

Common physical and emotional changes: These are the

following:

- Fetal movement is noticeable.
- There is no nausea during this stage.
- Mask of pregnancy (chloasma) may appear.
- Usually become constipated.
- Have food cravings.
- Sometimes develop vaginitis.
- There is usual problem of nasal congestion.
- Have leg cramps frequently.
- Change in voice.
- Painful groin from round ligament contractions.
- Weight gain.
- Pregnancy becomes more enjoyable.
- Sexual desires may change.

(Third trimester)

Fetal growth: Reaches to about 20 inches. Fingernails protrude beyond fingers. The head is large as compared to body. The arms and legs are in flexed position. Lungs become mature.

Placental and uterine changes: Uterus is back to height at 34th week. Placenta with one inch thickness have 6 to 8 inches diameter. Umbilical cord having length of approximately 20 to 22 inches (sometimes ranges between 12 to 39 inches also) has twisted or spiral appearance.

Common physical and emotional changes: Contractions, bloody show, progressive effacement and dilation, backache, ruptured membranes and loose bowel movements are some of the signs of labor.

(Postpartum care of child and mother)

- Newborn needs 10 to 20 hours sleep.
- Touching, cuddling and skin contact required.
- Uterine is at the height of navel after the birth and returns to pre-pregnant location and size by 10 days postpartum.
- After-pains in uterus are common and there is no need to worry.
- Urination and perspirations increases.
- Lochia (vaginal flow) is present.
- Breasts enlarge in case of breastfeeding.
- Fatigue and excitement exist.
- Weight loss may be 6 to 8 kg in early postpartum.
- The menstruation general does not return for months if breastfeeding, otherwise periods start in 4 to 8 weeks.
- Ovulation may be delayed, but is possible within weeks.
- Sexual relationship is readjusted and contraception.

9

Important Tips During Pregnancy

What to do in case of leakage of milk during pregnancy?

Breasts are felt hard, sore and soaked because of milk secretion from breasts in early or mid pregnancy often in the morning. Consult a gynecologist who will teach you how to take care of the breasts during pregnancy. Give a firm support to the breasts using a good quality and correct-sized brassier to match the cups, which should be loose and supportive, but not tight. Light exercises for the breast keep breast disorders at bay.

Is sex during pregnancy advisable?

Having sexual intercourse during pregnancy will not harm the fetus. One may continue sexual intercourse right up to the onset of labor. As the abdomen enlarges, a woman may find intercourse more comfortable in positions that put less or absolutely no pressure on abdomen like side-by-side or the female on the top. If you have complications like bleeding or pain in abdomen, refrain from sexual activity and even nipple stimulation is to be avoided in such cases as it can induce pre-term labor.

Doctors often advise to avoid intercourse from 6th to 12th week of pregnancy as it can cause miscarriage. Sexual abstinence is recommended during the last two months of pregnancy too. At this time, there is risk of the essential amniotic fluid leakage during intercourse. However, the couple can and should engage in gentle love making, fondling and kissing. Intercourse during the first three months and the last two months of pregnancy is not advisable. During 4th to 7th month of pregnancy, intercourse is allowed unless there are medical reasons. Sexual act such as oral and anal sex should be strictly avoided throughout the pregnancy.

What is 4-D ultrasound?

A 4-D Ultrasound is the latest addition in the armamentarium of an obstetrician. A 3-D Ultrasound gives a 3-D dimensional view of the baby in womb. An ultrasound gives a 2D dimensional view, which makes the diagnosis of the malformations and the surface of the body of baby and internal malformations can be visualized clearly. A 3-D Ultrasound is like a still photograph whereas a 4-D Ultrasound is like taking video film of fetus malformation and the pregnancy, especially in case the mother is over the age of 35 years and has delivered a malformed baby in past.

Rashes or pain on breasts

Rashes on the breast can be due to various reasons. The most common cause is due to the allergy by wearing synthetic brassiere or due to bacterial viral or fungal infection. A mammogram or an ultrasound is done in case of lumpy, painful breasts. If there is cyst in the breasts, you can take any analgesic and wear tight bras to support them and relieve pain. 400mg of vitamin E or B taken over a period of time may lessen the pain. If the pain is severe, danazol or hormone therapy is recommended. Periodic examination of breasts is also necessary.

Stretch marks on abdomen and stomach

Stretch marks on abdomen and stomach are common in women generally during pregnancy and after delivery of child. Striae gravidarum or stretch marks appear on the lower abdomen in 50 to 90 percent of all pregnant women usually in the later half of pregnancy. These may also appear on thighs, hips, buttocks, breasts and upper arms of women, which appear as pinkish lines on fair complexioned women and lighter than the normal skin in dark complexioned women. The market is flushed with creams and ointments to cure these stretch marks. The stretch marks depend upon the family history, weight gain and nutritional status.

Cramps and pain in abdomen during pregnancy

Between 30 to 50% women suffer cramps pain during or before menses, which differs from woman to woman . Persistent night cramps are often caused by poor circulation. The cramp felt in abdomen before menses are difficult to cope but doesn't show that there is any abnormality in the genitals of the woman. About 10% women pass through severe pain and cramps during menses and are even unable to walk due to stress and strain as in case of delivery of child. During menstruation the pain in the lower back and pelvis is common and is called as 'initial pain'. The main reason for such pain is due to hormonal changes generally as a result of the contraction of uterus when it discharges blood. Yogic exercises stimulating the nerves of affected part of legs relieve cramps. There are several natural remedies to cure this painful disorder as below:

- Add 7 drops of essential oil of aromatic spicy herb cloves to a teaspoon of sunflower oil and massage the muscles of affected area.
- Tincture of myrrh rubbed directly into the affected muscle, gives quick relief.
- Mix two drops of each of the essential oils of lemon, pine and juniper, and shake with 1 tablespoon of sunflower oil. Massage with the oil prior to exercise.

A hot water bath of the lower part of the abdomen relieves pain. Consult a doctor if the pain is severe and doesn't stop for few days. This pain is different from menstruation pain or a pain experienced during and after intercourse. Smoking, sleeplessness and taking carbohydrates and fatty foods worsen conditions. Bad sitting posture, frequent headache, diarrhea, constipation, nausea or pains prior to menstruation further worsen the condition.

Is morning sex permissible during pregnancy?

Early morning is the best time to have sex due to the following reasons:

- The testoterone level in male partner is higher in early morning hours.
- Men and women have higher levels of growth of the hormones due to increased energy after the restful night.
- Often a man awakes with a full bladder, which compresses the venous blood return and prevents blood escaping from the penis as a result the male partner experience spontaneous erections in the morning.
- Sex during the night when the blood flow to the digestive system is predominant lacks pleasure. Good sex act requires good blood flow towards sex organs and is achieved better in the morning with empty stomach.

Is ovary cancer is common in women due to frequent childbirth?

Yes, it is due to rapid succession of childbirth resulting in wear and tear of the cervical tissue and natural genital secretions. The following symptoms are observed when patient suffers from cervical cancer:

- Abnormal blood stained vaginal discharge.
- Intermittent prolonged menstrual bleeding.
- Intercourse bringing on bleeding.
- Foul smelling vaginal secretion.
- Pain in the lower abdomen.

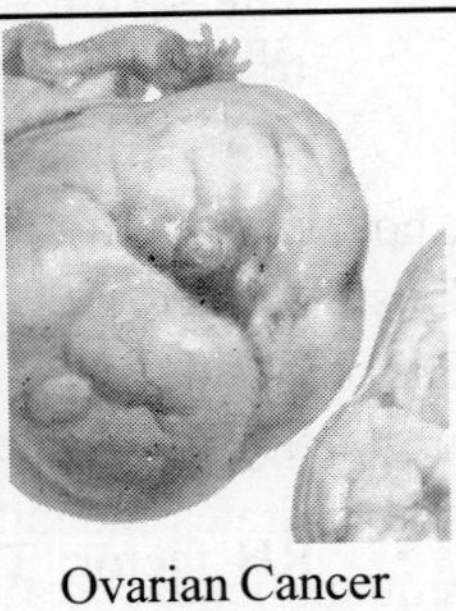

Ovarian Cancer

- Constant backache.
- Wear and tear of cervical tissues.

To treat cancer of cervix, measures such as surgical removal of affected part and destroying cancerous cells by radium or cobalt are adopted. If not treated at initial stage the cancerous cells may spread to liver and the brain.

Essential blood tests for a woman during pregnancy

A blood test could reveal various disorders in a woman's body. Every female from a pre-teen to a menopausal stage will at some time or the other have to undergo a blood test on the recommendation of doctor. The blood tests suggested for women are usually of six types:

- CBC-ESR test: is required to find out the presence of an infection or an inflammatory reaction. The test may count red cells in the blood. A high white blood count reveals the dreaded cancer of blood (Leukemia).
- Follicular stimulating Hormones (FSH) Test: This test is recommended to the teenage girls by the gynecologist in case of irregular periods.
- Haemogram: Women with excessive bleeding are required to go for Haemogram test, which highlights anemic condition and to check diabetes.
- The Serum Beta (HCG Blood) Test: The test is carried out to confirm pregnancy and is recommended when the woman has missed her periods.
- HIV Test: It is compulsory for every pregnant to examine sexually transmitted diseases such as Syphilis, Gonorrhea and Hepatitis-B, and to make a decision whether to continue the pregnancy.
- RH factor: The test is essential for pregnant women. If

the mother is RH negative (RH-) the baby is usually delivered through a caesarean procedure.

Pre-elcamptic toxemia in women

Pre-elcamptic toxemia (PET) is a combination of oedema (e.g. swelling on the ankles and fingers followed by puffiness of the face and with increased blood pressure and presence of protein in the urine). Obese women and teenage girls are usually seen suffering from this disorder. Women with family history of high blood pressure are prone to the risk. In case it is not treated timely there may be serious conditions of fits and the birth of a retard child due to infra-uterine growth affecting the growth of the infant in womb. The disease is more common in anemic and malnourished women. For a healthy growth of unborn baby, it is important to part with smoking and alcohol. Certain conditions like high blood pressure, chronic kidney diseases, heart ailments and some infections also affect baby's growth.

Nausea and vomiting

Nausea and vomiting are referred as 'morning sickness'. Pregnant women frequently feel nauseated and need to vomit when they have not eaten for several hours or when they smell some odors such as cigar smoke or certain foods being cooked. A woman may worry about her baby's health if she vomits frequently. A medical survey indicates that women healthy at the time of conception have sufficient reserves to supply the growing embryo and fetus even though they eat less. The following treatment recommended:

- Try to modify eating habits.
- Include sufficient protein in each of the meals.
- Eat crackers or toast before getting up in the morning.
- Drink liquids between instead of during meals.
- Increase intake of vitamin B 6 (Pyridoxine).

- Have a sense of humor.
- Medications are available to help control nausea and vomiting. Better consult your doctor.

Heartburn

Heartburn – a feeling of fullness is a common complaint in late pregnancy caused by combination of hormonal effects that relax the muscular opening, cause the stomach to empty more slowly and increase pressure from the growing uterus. Fatty foods, foods that produce gas and large meals may contribute to the condition. The following treatment is recommended:

- Avoid fatty foods and foods that produce gas.
- Eat several small meals and eat slowly.
- Do not eat just before bedtime.
- Use anti-acid or other drugs to control heartburn.

Constipation

During pregnancy the movement of food through the intestines is slowed due to pressure from the growing uterus on the large intestine magnifies the problem. Drink plenty of fluids. Eat foods with high fiber content such as raw or dried fruits, vegetables, whole grains and prune juice. Exercise regularly. Preventing constipation also alleviates the discomfort of hemorrhoids during pregnancy.

Sudden pain in the back that moves towards the right shoulder

It is common during pregnancy and generally starts in the night when pain suddenly starts inn the back and radiates to the right shoulder. To get relief, press the stomach. Sometimes, this pain may be due to accumulation of acidity in gall bladder. In case the pain is due to liver or kidney a complete bed rest is advised.

Rh factor in blood

There are hardly 10% women who have Rh factor in blood. In case of Rh negative female getting married to Rh positive male, her children can be either Rh negative or positive. If the fetus is Rh positive, the mother's system produces antibodies to protect her infant's Rh positive blood. This may lead to jaundice in the baby or a severe complication called erythroblastosis foetalis (severe anemia accompanied by jaundice). The pregnant woman's blood should be tested for Rh negative antibodies.

Pain in stomach and lower belly

Mild stomach or liver pain during pregnancy is not a matter of worry and is usually caused due to increased weight of the embryo and mother's nerves getting stained. Massage the stomach lightly with ghee to get relief. Constant pain in lower belly should be brought to the notice of doctor. A weak pregnant woman may have several abdominal discomforts during early pregnancy due to infection in pelvic organs or urinary tract.

A drop or two of blood oozing from uterus

This problem usually develops during 4th and 5th month from the date of conception and sometimes may lead to miscarriage. There is a small membrane in the uterus filled with amniotic fluid in which the fetus develops. In some cases the membrane gets swollen and the placenta orifice gets closed due to inflammation. This leads to the placenta puffing up and blood mixed with water accumulates in the region.

Severe itching, pain in vagina after intercourse

It could be either due to semen remaining in the vagina after intercourse or abrasion in the vaginal tract caused due to friction. It is suggested to avoid frequent sex during early stage of conception. If possible avoid frequent intercourse during the entire period of pregnancy as it may harm the child. The itching and the pain may spread to the anus also. Better have suggestion of a doctor.

Sudden increase in weight and swelling of body

Signs like sudden increase in weight, swelling of body, rise in blood pressure, appearance of albumin in urine, severe breathing trouble, constant thumping of heart and abrupt bleeding are warning signs that something is wrong with the pregnancy. Go for immediate medical advice. The pregnant woman must have a periodical check on weight, blood pressure and urine. A woman should not put more than 10 kg of weight during the entire period of pregnancy. There is often an increase of weight from the 3rd month onward, except the couple of weeks when there is hardly any increase in weight. Take a low salt but high protein diet.

Weakness, insomnia and exhaustion during pregnancy

Feeling too week and exhausted, loss of sleep (insomnia) especially during night, a constant tension, loss of appetite and constant fever are common disorders among women during pregnancy because of growing embryo. The following home remedies can alleviate the problems:

- Mix 2 parts each of pumpkin oil and poppy seed oil to I part of camphor and massage the head daily in the morning and evening.
- Massage the head with Brahmi or Narayan or Mahanarayan oil.
- Take Sarpagandatvaka Churan mixed in hot milk during night for a sound sleep.

Piles

Piles generally develop due to faulty food habits, irregular bowel routine, taking spicy foods and as a result of constipation, which irritate the stomach and intestines. In pregnant, piles usually develop due to abdominal pressure. It is better to maintain proper Bowel habits. Early cases of piles are treated with local anesthetics and ointments. In severe cases pile masses are pricked with syringes to shrink them. In some cases, piles develop a couple of months after the delivery. If the problem develops immediately after childbirth an anti-haemorrhoid ointment is recommended.

How to have a pregnancy test?

Most of the pregnancy tests are based on hormonal concentration of bHCG in urine. This test is sensitive and become positive as early as 2 to 3 days before missed period due to pregnancy. The accuracy is 98.5%. Collect the early morning urine sample in a clean bottle. Only a few drops of urine are sufficient for a pregnancy test. 14 days after a missed period is the usual time to have a pregnancy test. A few doctors suggest hormone pills. Sometimes, a woman may bleed even if she is pregnant and this delays the finding out sure pregnancy.

When a woman is willing for a abortion

Women with unwanted pregnancies always resort to abortion. With restricted law imposed by the Government, an abortion is illegal. The pregnancy may be due to the following reasons:

- Contraceptive failure.
- Act of an intercourse when got drunk in late night parties in higher society and fairly liberal families, which sometimes end with sex.
- Strong mutual attraction towards opposite sex.
- Effect of sexy TV serials and movies.
- Too shy to discuss contraception with the male partner, when a female becomes pregnant.
- Urge to have sex with opposite sex in youth without thinking about its after-effect.

- Fulfill the desire of boss at the place of work.
- Desire to have more money.
- Bad society in youth.

Most abortions are carried out before 12 weeks of pregnancy and by the common method called vacuum aspiration or suction. The cervix is dilated or widened carefully and the contents of the womb are sucked out using a suction apparatus.

Another method of abortion, instead of vacuum aspiration between 12 to 14 weeks of pregnancy is dilation and curettage by inserting prostaglandin pessaries (a thimble -like fine rubber cervical cap about 15 cm. long, which looks like a condom used by males, can be pushed into the vagina to cover the external genitalia and uterine mouth prior to coitus and should be slipped out 5 to 6 hours after the intercourse. The use of pessary combined with a spermicidal cream is more effective. Another substance called laminaria is also inserted into the vagina to avoid pregnancy.

The contents of the womb are removed by instrument called a curette made of soft wire rather than by section. It cleans the womb and most of the tissues removed during abortion look like a very heavy period. If the bleeding persist and is very heavy, consult a doctor immediately. Retained products in uterus lead to an infection. This sometimes happen about a week or ten days after the abortion.

Abortion after 12 weeks

It becomes more difficult although it is still a safe technique. In this process instead, after dilating the cervix, the doctor may insert instruments into the womb. The technique is called dilation and evacuation and is carried out under general anesthesia. Late abortions are conducted by hysterectomy, a technique used very rarely, which involves removing contents of the womb in an operation very like a caesarean section. It is done under general anesthetic.

Any abortion conducted after 12 weeks is likely to cause pain and cramps, which may last several days and the womb shrinks back to its pre-pregnancy size. The bleeding will also go on for about a week. Avoid activities like swimming, soaking in a hot bath, wearing tampon or having sexual intercourse for six weeks.

A regular practice of exercises to strengthen the reproductive organs makes pregnancy strong and a healthy fetus. Premature delivery is common in women in which usually the infant is delivered in the eight month and doesn't survive in 75% cases. This is due to the weakness of cervical muscles, which support the uterus in expectant mother and suffer miscarriage.

Do's and don'ts about breast care and breastfeeding

- Keep breast nipples clean and dry to prevent them from becoming sore and infected. Do not apply soap to clean nipples and areola to avoid cracks.
- Wash breasts and nipples with water to remove traces of milk.
- Make sure to change bra frequently. The secretion of nipples causes infection.
- In case nipples are not soft and supple, apply some cream or oil. Avoid use of mustard oil, it is irritates. Keep breasts exposed to air for sometime in a day.
- Prevent engorgement of breasts to ensure frequent emptying and after a feed.
- Breasts sag if the infant suckles while sitting or reclining in a faulty posture. Always let the baby suckles in a sitting position with the child in the lap and mother's hands under the head.
- Remove the remaining milk with a couple of jerks after feeding the child.

Importance of breast milk

Breast-feeding is the most perfectly balanced food that a baby needs for growth during first 3-4 months. It prevents many illness, infections and allergies. Lactation helps in controlling the bleeding after the delivery, the womb returns to its normal position, sheds extra weight gained during the pregnancy, prevents cancer and helps in spacing children. Breastfeeding is very convenient for mother during travel and the milk is more digestible as compared to cow's milk.

10

Warning Signs During Pregnancy

During pregnancy, report any of the following warning signs to your doctor:

Warning Signs		Possible Problems
Vaginal bleeding	:	Miscarriage, Placenta previa, Abruptio placenta, Premature labour.
Abdominal pain	:	Ectopic pregnancy, Abruptio placenta, Early labor contractions.
Leaking or gushing of fluid from vagina	:	Rupture of the membranes.
Puffiness or swelling of hands, feet, face	:	Pre-eclampsia (toxemia).
Severe, persistent headache	:	Pre-eclampsia (toxemia).
Vision disturbance, blind spots and flashes	:	Pre-eclampsia (toxemia).
Dizziness, light headedness, hypotensio	:	Pre-eclampsia or supine hypotension.
Pain or burning on urination	:	Urinary tract infection, Sexually transmitted disease.

Irritating vaginal discharge, sores, itching	:	Vaginal infection and STD.
Fever (oral temperature)	:	Infection.
Persistent nausea or vomiting	:	Hyperemesis gravidarum and infection.
Noticeable reduction in fetal activity	:	Fetal distress.

Perineal massage for painless delivery

Perineal massage has different purpose than most massage. It is used to soften the tissue around the vagina, relax pelvic floor muscles and increase the elasticity of the perineum by taking advantage of the hormonal changes that loosen connective tissue in the late pregnancy when there is pressure before and during birth. A regular perineal massage (at least 6 to 8 weeks before due date) helps avoiding an episiotomy or a serious tear during childbirth. Remember, if you have vaginitis, herpes or other vaginal problem, be sure to get checked before beginning perineal massage as it could worsen the condition. You can do self-massage or seek the help of your partner. Wash your hands before massaging. Be sure that your fingernails are short. If the skin of hands is rough, wear disposable rubber gloves. Sit in a comfortable semi-sitting position squatting against a wall or sitting on the toilet. The following procedure should be adopted while doing perineal massage:

- Lubricate your fingers with oil or water-soluble jelly (K-Y jelly). Wheat-germ oil is recommended as it contains high vitamin E content. Do not use mineral oil or petroleum jelly. Wash your hand every time before dipping into lubricant.

- Rub enough oil or jelly into the perineum to allow your fingers move smoothly over the tissue and lower vaginal wall.

- You may use your thumb during self-massage or your partner can use his index finger. Put the fingers or thumb well inside the vagina up to the second knuckle, move them upward along the sides of the vagina in a rhythmic U or sling-type movement to help stretching the vaginal tissue (mucosa), muscles around vagina and smoothen skin of the perineum by rubbing between the thumb and forefinger.
- Concentrate on relaxing your muscles as you apply pressure comfortably.
- Massage for about five minutes.

How to strengthen pelvic floor muscles?

The pelvic floor or perineal muscles act as a support for your abdominal and pelvic organs, which usually sag during pregnancy due to increased weight of your uterus and the relaxing effect of the hormones produced by your body. A regular exercise of the pelvic floor muscles (which forms a figure 8, circling around the urethra, vagina and anus) maintain tone, improve circulation and reduce the heavy, throbbing feeling that you might experience during pregnancy or post partum. A regular exercise of the pelvic floor is important during pregnancy and as well as throughout your lifetime, which also increase sexual enjoyment for you and your partner. Problems such as leakage of urine and relaxation of the rectal wall can also be prevented or reduced if the muscle of pelvic floor is maintained. To check the strength of your pelvic floor muscles, try to stop the flow of urine in midstream. You may also check by inserting two fingers in the vagina and tightening your pelvic floor muscles around them. At the time of intercourse, check by tightening your pelvic floor muscles around your partner's genital organ (penis). The following exercise movements are suggested:

- **Pelvic floor contraction (Perineal squeeze or Kegal exercise):** maintains the tone of the pelvic floor muscles, improves circulation to the perineum. Contract or tighten the pelvic muscles as if you would stop the flow of urine. Hold tightly for 2-3 seconds, release tension, relax and lower pelvic floor. Repeat several times.

- **Squatting:** increase the mobility of the pelvic joints, stretch the muscles and ligaments of the inner thighs and calves. It eases delivery of child. Slowly squat with your weight on your whole foot, not just your toes as if you are sitting for toilet. Stay down for 30 seconds to two minutes at a time, then rise slowly.

- **Abdominal tightening**: strengthen and tone the abdominal muscles. Sit up with your hands on your abdomen. Breathe in allowing your abdomen to bulge. As you breathe out, gradually tighten your abdominal muscles by pulling in your abdomen towards your backbone until your lungs are empty. Repeat 2-3 times.

- **Pelvic tilt**: strengthen the abdominal muscles, improve posture and relieve backache. Lie on your back with your knees bent and feet flat on the floor. Flatten the small of your back onto the floor by contracting abdomen muscles five times.

- **Pelvic rocking**: Move on your hands and knees, keeping your back straight.

- **Leg sliding**: strengthen the lower abdominal muscles. Lie on your back with knees bent and feet flat on the floor. Put your hand beneath the small of your back. Maintain a pelvic tilt with your lower back flat against your hand while slowing sliding your feet straightening both legs until you feel your low back come up.

- **Stretching:** helps increase flexibility and promotes comfort during pregnancy and childbirth. Sit on the floor with your knees bent and soles of your feet together. Lean forward from your hips, relaxing your legs. Allow the weight of your legs to stretch muscles of the inner thighs, outer thighs and buttocks gently pressing your knees toward the floor. Repeat this exercise for three to four times.

- **Hamstring stretch**: stretch the hamstring muscles (at the back of thighs) to help relieve backache. Sit on the floor extending your left leg straight out. Touch your left foot with both hands keeping your back straight. Repeat on the other leg.
- **Calf stretch**: stretch the tendons and muscles of the calf and ankle. Slowly and gently bend your front knee, putting your weight onto the front leg keeping back straight. Hold for 30-60 seconds. Then repeat on other leg. Repeat 3-4 times.

Why and when miscarriage takes place?

A miscarriage or spontaneous abortion is the unexpected and involuntary expulsion of the embryo or fetus before the 20th week of pregnancy. Occasionally, a miscarriage occurs because of an acute infection, a severe physical shock, an imbalance of hormones, a defective ovum or sperm and faulty intrauterine environment. The signs of a possible miscarriage are vaginal bleeding and intermittent pain, which usually begins in the lower back and is later felt as abdominal cramping.

Pre-natal examination ?

Prenatal examination or care helps assure the birth of a healthy baby. The following tests and examinations are performed at the prenatal visits:

- A complete medical history and physical examination of expectant mother.
- A pelvic (vaginal) examination to estimate the size and shape of your pelvis, to confirm pregnancy, to do a Pap smear to detect cervical cancer and to test for venereal disease such a syphilis and gonorrhea.

- A complete blood test to determine your blood type, Rh factor, to test for anemia, blood sugar, infection and German measles immunity.
- Weight check, blood pressure, urine tests for diabetes and to detect excess protein.
- Abdominal examination to measure the growth of the uterus (fundal height), growth of the fetus and estimate the size and position of the fetus.

11

Genital Diseases During Pregnancy

There are following diseases related to female genital organs concerning vulva, vagina and the cervix, which may harm pregnancy:

DISEASES OF VULVA

Bartholin's Glands

A vulva disease, causing abscesses or cysts due to infection during reproductive years including pregnancy with the signs and symptoms:

- Painful swelling of labia.
- Formation of abscess or on vagina.
- Clear or yellow or blue cysts at the base of the labia majora.

To prevent the disease Avoid or reduce exposure to sexually transmitted diseases and vulva trauma.

Contact Vulvitis

Vulva irritation during pregnancy caused by the following factors:

- Severe irritation.
- Un-hygienic conditions most common during pregnancy.

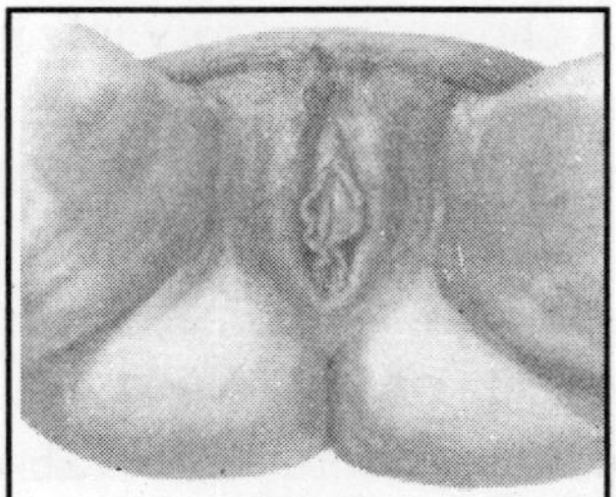

Contact Vulvitis

- Ill-effect of deodorants and soaps used on genital area.
- Wearing tight-fitting and synthetic under-garments, tampons or pads, perfumes, scented toilet paper, laundry soap.
- Effect of condoms, lubricants, topical contraceptives and sexual aids used during pregnancy.
- When frequent vaginal secretions during pregnancy or semen remains in the vagina for a long time.
- Soiling of vulva by urine or faces.

The signs and symptoms of this disorder include severe dermatitis of vulva, reddening of vulva skin accompanied by itching and burning, vulva dystrophy and excessive vaginal secretions.

Dysareunia Insertional

It is common in women during the pregnancy and the reproductive age. It is caused due to several factors such as inadequate lubrication in vaginal canal, phobias while having sex, pelvis muscle spasm, scarring in the vaginal canal, surgical repairs to the vulva and effect of herpes vulvitis. The disorder leads to severe burning or pinching. Treatment includes vaginal lubrication, regular practice of pelvic relaxation exercises techniques to reduce pain during intercourse and improved position during sexual intercourse.

Hidradenitis Suppurative

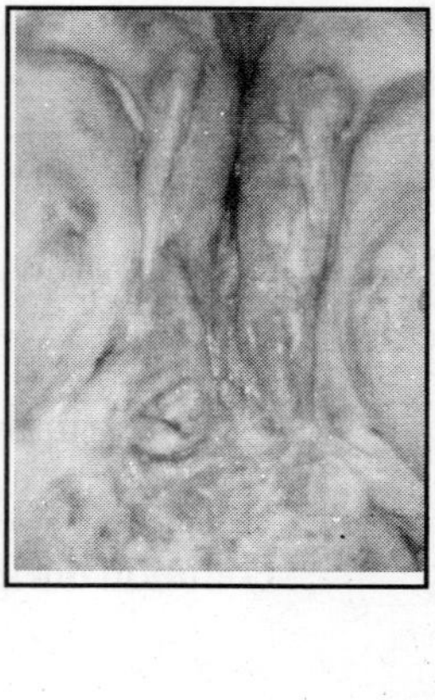

A chronic refractory infection of the skin and subcutaneous tissues causing inflammation and formation of abscess involving vulva and perineum. Other symptoms include recurrent inflammation on labia with severe pain, foul smelling discharge, formation of abscess and sexual transmitted disease.

General measures for the treatment of this disease are perineal hygiene, a Sitz's bath, administering antibiotics in consultation with a doctor, avoid formation of scarring, abscesses and infection.

Vulva Dystrophy

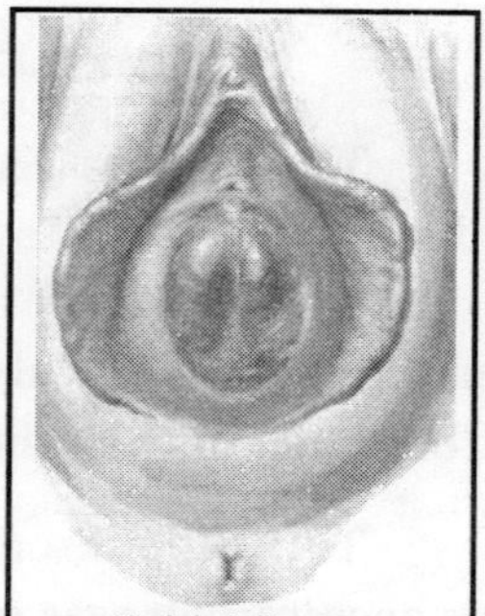

Initial Stage

Thickening of vulva skin over the labia majora, labia minora and clitorial areas accompanied with inflammation, irritation, itching, fissuring and excoriations. If not treated timely, the disease can cause cancer of the vulva and chronic vulvitis.To treat this disease the measures such as perineal hygiene, reducing stress, a Sitz's bath and reducing contact allergy are adopted. The patient should strictly follow precautions e.g. wear gloves during night to avoid tissue damages due to scratching and avoid itching and scratching.

Lichen Sclerosus

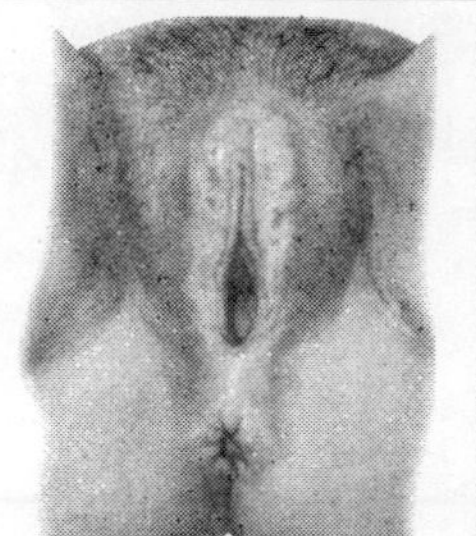

Lichen Sclerosus

It is a chronic condition causing vulva inflammation generally in pregnancy, late reproductive age and during early menopausal when there is intense itching, scratch marks or fissures around the anus. Perineal hygiene, a Sitz's bath and application of petroleum jelly and some of the measures to treat this disorder If not treated timely, complications such as cancer of vulva, scarring and narrowing of the vaginal canal resulting in surgical delivery may arise.

Vulva Hematoma

The disease consists of swelling of one or both labia because of the following reasons:

- Interstitial bleeding occurring due to sexual intercourse or a rape during pregnancy.
- Effect of varicose veins of vulva.
- Hard labor activities.

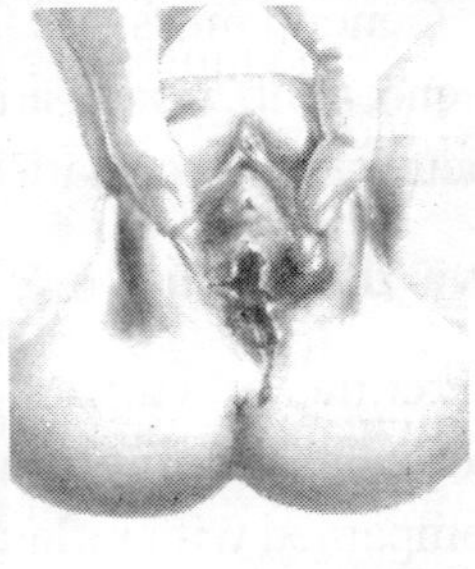
Vulvar Hematoma
Final Stage

The signs and symptoms of this disease are painful swelling of one or both labia, dark blue or black discoloration of vulva, bleeding and formation of cysts and abscess.

To treat the disorder, apply ice packs on vulva. Surgical drainage is necessary in case of rapidly expanding symptoms.

VAGINAL DISEASES

Cystocele and Urethrocele

A vaginal disease caused by lack of support due to ruptured vagina, pro-lapse of the urethra or bladder due to loss of normal tissue integrity caused by previous surgical childbirth or a obstetric injury, pressure on the pelvic region, urinary infections, formation of cysts, tumors and abscess on urethra.

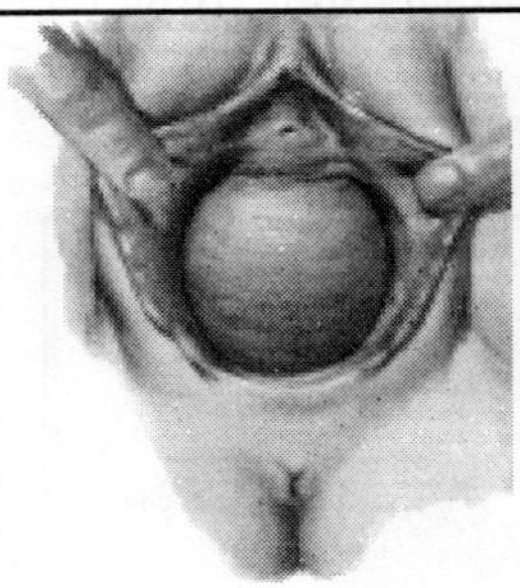
Large Cystocele

The following measures are advised to treat this disorder:

- Weight-reduction.
- Pelvic muscle exercises.
- Surgical repairs.
- Avoiding heavy lifting and straining.

- Consult a doctor immediately in case vaginal bleeding and symptoms of breast cancer.

Rectocele

It is due to failure of the normal support mechanism between the rectum and the vagina due to childbirth, obesity, heavy lifting and weakness of intrinsic tissue. The main signs and symptoms of this disease are bulging of posterior vaginal wall, difficulty in passing stool, risk of a rectal cancer, vaginal cyst and uterine pro-lapse. Weight loss, systemic estrogen replacement, pelvic muscle exercises and surgical repair are some of the measures to treat this disorder.

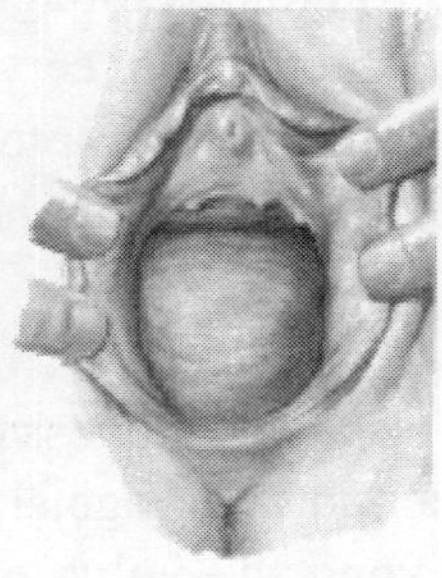

Large Rectocele

Vaginal Cysts

A common disorder in females from adolescence to middle reproductive years generally caused due to factors e.g. episiotomy (vaginal cut) in previous delivery and gynecologic surgery. Cystic lesions ranging up to 5 cm. are found in the lateral vaginal wall. Surgical excision is the only reliable treatment.

Vaginal Dryness

Loss of normal vaginal moisture causing irritation, itching and pain during sexual intercourse and inflamed vaginal tissue are prominent signs and symptoms of this disorder. Vaginal dryness occurs due to inadequate or inappropriate sexual stimulation, sexual phobia or pain more common in pregnant or menopausal women. Some prominent measures to treat such dryness are topical moisturizing, lubrication of vagina, estrogen replacement therapy and use of water- soluble lubricants before intercourse. If not treated properly, it may lead to vaginal lacerations, infections, vulva excoriations and sexual dysfunction.

Vaginal Laceriation

It is caused due to frequent sexual intercourse during pregnancy usually under the influence of alcohol and drugs causing injury and penetration by foreign objects. Vaginal bleeding, persistent pain after the intercourse, cervical polyp, bleeding and threatened abortion are signs and symptoms of this disorder. To treat it, have pelvic rest and avoid sex until healing occurs.

Vaginal Pro-lapse

It occurs due to loss of normal support to fetus resulting in vaginal wall-down in vaginal canal when in extreme cases vagina is displaced beyond the vulva outside the body. Frequent childbirth, intra-abdominal pressure, heavy lifting and intrinsic tissue weakness is the prominent causes of vaginal pro-lapse. Regular pelvic pain, uterus dyspareunia, bleeding and vaginal cyst or tumor is sign and symptoms of this disorder.

Bacterial Vaginitis

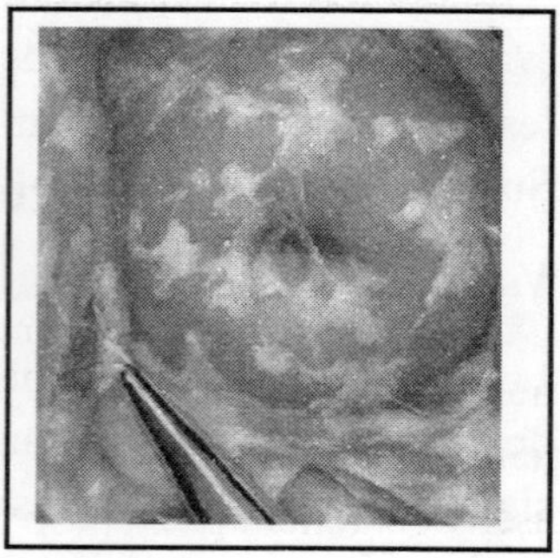

A vaginal infection caused by excessive growth of bacteria causes severe itching, irritation and inflammation in genital area in females between the age of 15 to 50, generally during pregnancy due to suffering from diabetes, pregnancy and debilitating disease, habit of too much smoking, frequent intercourse during pregnancy, effect of excess number of sexual partners, too much use of vaginal contraceptives, oral sex, and unhygienic conditions especially during pregnancy. Perineal hygiene is an important measure to treat this disorder. If neglected, the possible complications like cystitis, cervicitis, severe infections, pelvic inflammatory disease, pelvic pain, infertility, increased risk of upper genital- tract infection, premature delivery and premature rupture of the membranes may take place. An pregnant should immediately seek the consultation of a gynecologist.

Vaginitis-Monilial

A vaginal infection caused by fungi found in the atmosphere at vagina, rectum and vaginal mouth usually occurs in female between15 to 50 years age generally during the period of pregnancy due to frequent secretions. Nearly 80 to 90 % cases of this vaginal disease are caused due to candida albicus, candida glabrata or candida tropicals.

Avoid stress, diabetes, depression, topical contraceptives and warm and moist environments.

The patients face symptoms such as vulva itching or burning, scratching, edema, vulva excoriations, white to yellow thick pussy discharge and pinworms. Following are the important measures to treat the disease. Perineal hygiene and keeping the affected area clean and dry are the main precautions taken by the patient. Avoid wearing tight synthetic undergarments and topical steroid preparations.

Vaginitis Trichomonas

A vaginal infection common in pregnant females caused by too much sex, vaginal pH (less acid in blood and semen) causing vulva itching or burning and thin runny yellow to green to gray foul odor discharge. If not treated properly, it leads to complications like cystitis (inflammation of the bladder resulting in frequent urge to pass urine), pain in lower abdomen, pelvic inflammation and pelvic pain. This disorder can be cured by medical treatment. Consult a doctor immediately.

DISEASES OF CERVIX

Intra-epithelia Lesion

It consists of carcinoma in cervical generally in reproductive age or during pregnancy. Vaginitis, cervicitis and cervical dysplasia are the main symptoms. Consult your doctor for treatment. Pap smears examination, cryo-therapy,. Electro-cautery and electro-surgical loop excision are the required treatments. But these are very harmful during pregnancy.

Carcinoma in Cervix

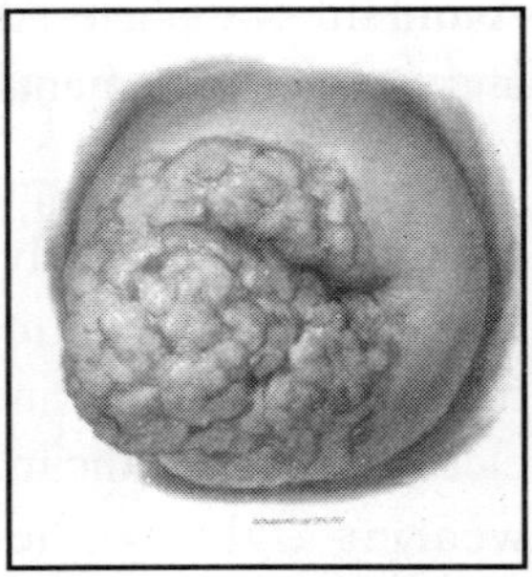

The thickness of epithelium is replaced with invasive carcinoma usually occur during pregnancy. The prominent causes of this disorder are herpes virus, early sexual activities, too much or multiple sexual partners, use of oral contraceptives and early childbearing. The measures to treat the disease are standard hysterectomy, ablative therapy, cryosurgery and CO2 laser therapy. Seek advice of a doctor as these treatments are very harmful for pregnant women.

Cervical Cancer

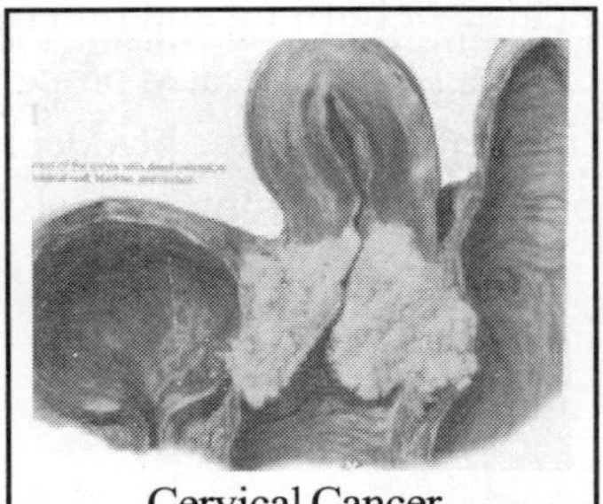

Cervical Cancer

Almost all cancers of cervix are carcinoma. The disease is often seen in women during pregnancy and is generally caused due to early sexual activities, too much or multiple sex partners and presence of sexually transmitted viral infections. Signs and symptoms of the disease include abnormal Pap smear, vaginal bleeding, dark vaginal discharge, loss of appetite, weight loss, bleeding lesion, inguinal lymph nodes, swelling of legs, cervical erosion and cervical polyp. Chemotherapy is curative measure to treat the disease, but seek advice of a doctor for treatment.

Cervical Erosion

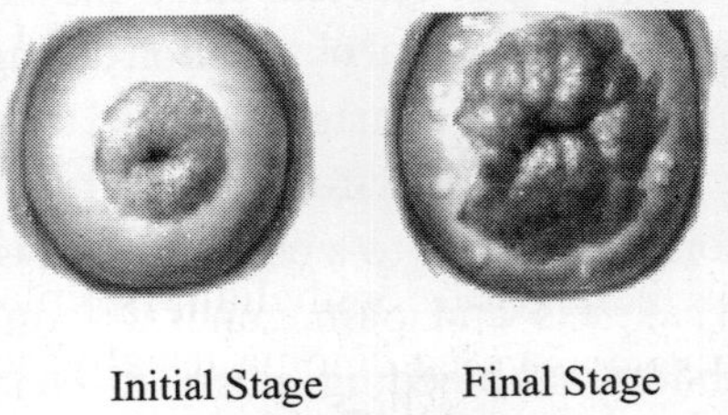

Cervical Erosions

Loss of epithelial on vaginal portion due to the fingernails to relieve irritation and frequent itching during pregnancy are the prominent causes of this disorder. The signs and symptoms of disease include suffering from syphilis, irregularly shaped lesions, bleeding tissues, spotting, increased vaginal discharge, herpes simplex and carcinoma under the epithelium surface.

Cervical Polyps

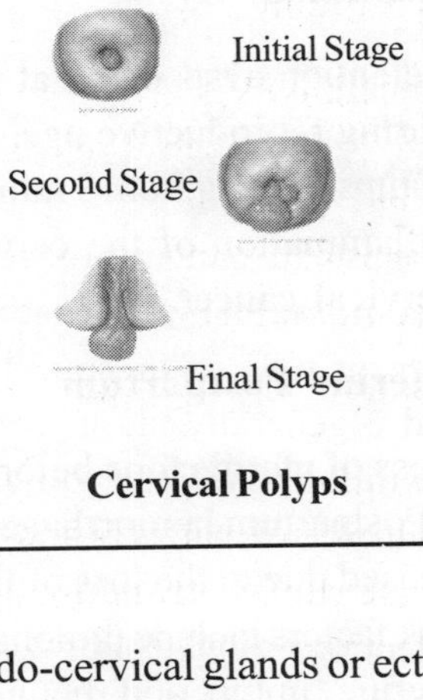

Cervical Polyps

Fleshy tumors arising from the cells of cervix generally in the age group of 40 t0 50 in women having history of cervical infections and use of oral contraceptives, resulting in frequent inflammation. Symptoms include inter-mentrual spotting, post-coital spotting and reddish purple to cherry red friable mass up to 4 cm. size at cervix. A pap smear test is essential.

Cervicitis

Acute or ethronic inflammation of the endo-cervical glands or ectocervix, usually during reproductive age and sometimes in adolescence. It is caused by exposure to sexual infection, multiple sexual partners. Consult doctor for treatment immediately.

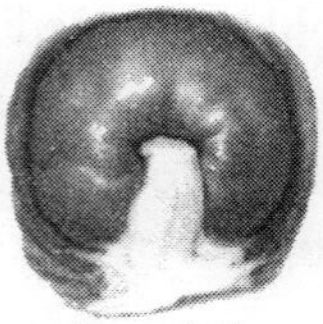

Appearance of cervix in acute infection

Cervical Stenosis

Narrowing of cervical canal may result in complete or partial obstruction during intercourse and childbirth when pregnant. The damage is caused by several reasons such as infection, cone-biopsy, electrocautery, cryocautery, radiation, infection and sometime due to congenital reasons, which cause a sense of weakness and pain generally due to irritation in the ovaries, abdominal bleeding, pussy discharge in pregnant women, scanty discharge of menstruation blood in young females, uterine enlargement.

To treat the disorder, mix black sesame seeds with equal quantity of small caltrops (gokhru) in 250 ml water. Grind, sweeten and drink. Dilation of the cervix under ultrasound guidance cures the disease.

Nabothian Cysts

Retention cysts occur at the closure of a gland opening generally during reproductive age. These are raised white to blue to yellow bumps ranging from 3 mm. to 3 cm. in diameter, which cause chronic inflammation of the cervix, followed by mucus-filled cysts and cervical cancer.

Uterine Postpartum

Loss of uterine tone before or after the delivery that often presents a Postpartum hemorrhage generally seen in about 5% cases, and is caused due to the loss of the normal uterine contractile forces. The risk factors include prolonged labor, prolonged oxytocin stimulation, uterine rupture and retained placental tissue in the uterus.

Signs and symptoms of this disorder include:

- Bright red vaginal bleeding.
- loss of uterine tone.

To treat this disorder, massage the uterus fundus and the bladder should be drained to allow the uterus to contract.

12

Planning for a Healthy Child?

Depression during pregnancy

Depression is common among pregnant women as well as after the childbirth, which causes a woman not only to lose sexual and other interests, besides feeling irritability and fatigue most of the time. The depression is more likely to occur if woman feels isolated and inadequate support from her husband and other members of her family. During the period of pregnancy, the mother should pay visits to the doctor for regular check up between six and eight weeks and also after delivery of the child, which gives the mother the opportunity to discuss any problem faced by her.

The following natural remedies are suggested:

- Sunlight: Body needs sunlight. The lack of sunlight can disturb the production of key hormones and brain chemicals triggering depression.
- Exercise: It is must to reduce depression. An hour a day of exercise for a week is universal prescription for depressed people.
- Light music: Music lifts depression.

Overweight

If you have started gaining weight during pregnancy, your tummy has put on extra flesh because of your skin and muscles must have grown to hold the constant weight of baby in womb. Do not worry, the muscles gradually start tighten up again some time after the childbirth. Do not forget to undertake gentle exercises during pregnancy after consulting your doctor. Breastfeeding helps the stomach to get back to shape as it helps the uterus to contract and within two months after the delivery, the uterus takes non-pregnant size.

How to plan for a healthy child?

Remember, child's health does not start after the birth, even before the baby is conceived in the mother's womb. Planning of a child must be considered in three factors: before conception, during conception and after conception during the period of pregnancy. Oral contraceptives have harmful side effects and are not advised. Start treatment under acupressure therapy at least three months prior to conceiving in the following ways:

- The couple should take a glass of charged water (health drink) daily.
- The female partner must have three regular menses before conceiving to have a healthy fully developed uterus.
- A daily massage on both sides of wrists for five minutes by female partner proves beneficial for a healthy pregnancy.

To prepare charged water (health drink), mix 300 gm. of Amla powder to 100 gm. ginger powder. Swallow one teaspoonful of this powder with water in the morning and evening. Another way is to add two teaspoonful of above powder of Amla and ginger in four glasses of water. Use fresh Amla and ginger (if available). Boil the mixture, till it is reduced to three glasses. Filter the liquid and add to it salt or honey to your taste. Amla is concentrated form of vitamin C. It has 16 times more vitamin C than lemon and helps to provide protection to the body against cold and increases digestion power. Health drink is beneficial especially for the convalescing people, old, growing children and the expectant mothers.

Acupressure Therapy

It is exceptionally beneficial for pregnant women. Nature has provided the body with proper regulators and protectors. These are our endocrine glands, which secrete hormones directly into our blood. The proper functioning of these glands is very important and most vital for good health for the development of our body, mind, looks and even character. Malfunctioning of endocrine glands adversely affect the reproductive organs in human body. Pineal gland, too, control sex system and water in the body, which leads to premature sex development. Malfunctioning of ovaries, testes and sex glands control heat of productive organs of body, which damage reproductive organs and cause problems of menstruation, self-abuse and lesser or more sex desire.

Apply pressure on the palms for healthy pregnancy. Here are few important tips to be kept in mind during, before and after conception, pregnancy and post-natal period:

- The couple must start treatment under acupressure therapy at least three months prior to conceiving.
- Ensure proper creation of hormones.
- Drink a glass of Health Drink (Gold/Silver/Copper/Iron charged water) every day.
- Ensure female partner must have three regular menses before conceiving.

How to have a healthy child?

According to Naturopathy, if the intercourse is conducted during the dates 10th to15th the day on which the menses is seen, there is better possibility of conceiving and the child to be born, if conceived, will be healthy. During the period of menstruation flow, the couple should avoid intercourse and if the conception occurs during this period, there is possibility of the child being born with physical and mental defects. You should keep in mind the following tips, which are essential to have a healthy baby:

- In case of problems, such as early, irregular, scanty, painful or excessive menstruation, the treatment of pressing points 11 to 15 on both wrists will leave amazing results to regulate menstruation and cure Leucorrhoea (white or yellow vaginal discharge accompanied by pus.
- During first pregnancy the expectant mother usually feel worried and have lot of tension, which adds to the labor pains vitally affecting both body and mind. Even in the case of the use of forceps or caesarean section (surgical operation) the child's body may get damaged and even the mother is hurt.
- To have a painless childbirth, roll grooved wooden roller vigorously on the back of both arms from nail to elbow for about 15 minutes. If roller is not available, rub palms and soles with two metal combs vigorously from nails to wrist for 5 to 10 minutes. For painless childbirth, apply continuous pressure on the back part of the tongue beyond the teeth for a minute and repeat few times with an interval of three minutes.
- To avoid difficult labor, press hard on the inner side above the ankles for two minutes. Pause and press again and again till the child is born. There is often severe pain after the birth of infant due to accumulation of milk in the breasts, which should be expressed after breastfeeding. Press on the middle portion of the back of both palms. It relieves breast pain and inflammation.

Few important points:

- After the delivery of the baby or operation for sterilization there is great possibility of the woman putting on fat because the sex glands are disturbed. Acupressure therapy helps a lot to relieve this problem. Press point No. 11 to 15 on the palms, which benefit in maintaining of good physique.

- Applying pressure on points 11 to 15 on palms help enough production of milk for the baby. This also cures impotency in males and frigidity in females.
- Men and women if disturbed by erotic dreams and get discharged (due to wet dreams) while in sleep, successfully try this natural treatment.
- In case of suffering from syphilis or other venereal diseases, massage ice on the affected part for two to four minutes a day according to the condition.
- Here is another treatment for those not suffering from diabetes. Take first urine and add to it one to two teaspoons of Soda bicarb. Boil the urine, allow it to cool, remove upper crust with cotton soaked in the urine and massage the affected part and area around it for five to six minutes. Now clean the area with an antiseptic liquid.

Have a child of desired sex

The couple will be in a position to have a child of desired sex if the day on which the menses is seen is to be counted as the first day. The couple should avoid sexual intercourse during menses. Otherwise if there is conception in this period, there is possibility of child born with physical and mental defects. According to naturopaths, the following tips are advised for getting a child of desired sex:

- For getting a male child, on the even dates such as 4, 6, 8, 10, 12, 14 day, the husband should lie with his wife on the left side during sleep for 15 minutes to enable him to breathe with his right nostril before they indulge in sexual intercourse.
- For getting a female child, it is suggested that on odd dates such as 5, 7, 9, 11, 13, 15 day the husband should lie with his wife on right side for 15 minutes to enable him to breathe with his nostril before preparing for sexual intercourse.
- If the intercourse is made during the later dates between

10th to 15th day after the first day of last menses, there is possibility of conceiving immediately and the child to be born will be healthy.

After the baby is conceived, the mother should take proper care about her nourishment as described below:

- Eat plenty of seasonal fruits and drink enough milk to get maximum natural calcium.
- The expectant mother should have acupressure therapy treatment.
- Should undertake light exercises including walking throughout pregnancy period to ensure healthy growth of baby in womb.
- Remember, the child starts learning from the mother's womb. The husband should keep his wife happy during the vital period of pregnancy.

Marriage in blood relations

It should be avoided as far as possible. Such marriages are genetically unhealthy as both husband and wife carry the same type of genes, which could intensify the unhealthy manifestation in the newly born child. of a married couple, both were suffering from diabetes. The first baby they had was mentally retarded. The couple had normal second baby and the third issue was a premature, died at birth. The fourth baby the mother delivered was diabetic since birth.

Cleaning genital organs

Cleanliness of genital organs is very essential for men and women. For having genital bath, take off your clothes. Sit on a stool in a water tub filled with cold water in summer and lukewarm water in winter. The level of water should be 1-2 inches above the organ to be washed. Take a piece of cloth in water and gently rub your abdomen for two minutes.

In case of men, take hold of the foreskin of male organ in two fingers and rub in lightly with soft piece of cloth dipping in cold water followed by rubbing the entire spine with a wet towel.

In case of women, they should rub their abdomen first as above. Then pull the lips of the vagina and rub slowly with a wet piece of cloth. In the end rub the spine. Genital bath as well as Hip Bath should not be taken at the time during menstruation. If the tub is not available, genital bath can be taken in the sun in the same way.

Why pregnancy causes cancer in women?

In women two most likely places where cancer may develop includes breasts and the uterus. Both areas can easily be examined. Every young woman should be taught to examine her own breasts after each menstrual period. In case of detection of a tumor or anything unusual, a woman should seek advice of a doctor. Any kind of abnormality or feeling of the breast tissue outlining the curves within the breasts and up in the armpit should be examined thoroughly. Cancer of the cervix, breast or uterus is most common in women. Over 40% females suffer from cervical cancer, nearly 12% from breast cancer and the remaining cancer patients are seen suffering from vaginal or cancer of the other parts of body.

Breast Tumor and Cancer: is very common in women of every age. If there is only one single nodule or lump in the breasts: painful or without pain, it should always be removed. In case the cancer appears to have extended into the neighboring lymph nodes, the patient should be given extensive radiation therapy. Majority of breast cancers occur in either the upper portion of the breast, towards the shoulder or close to the nipple. Breast cancer is more common in women between the age of 35 and 65 years. It may also occur in teenage girls.

Cancer in Cervix is a vicious killer of woman today. Every female after the age 18 should have a pelvic examination and a Pap smear at least once a year or after six months. Any pain in the lower belly or a water discharge should be investigated, as it could be a cancer. Be careful, if the bleeding or spotting follows intercourse or douching. Modern treatment for the uterine cancer consists of implanting a small amount of radium within the cervical canal followed later by heavy dose of radiation therapy to the whole area. Performing a hysterectomy, removing the uterus, cervix, ovaries and tubes are the common treatments performed when suffering from a cervical cancer.

Cancer in Uterus: is less common type of cancer, known as fundal carcinoma. It may sometimes develop within the cavity of uterus itself. This is less malignant than cancer of the cervix and can be detected by Pap smear. If cancer is found, a hysterectomy should be done without delay. The cancer cells find their way into the abdominal cavities and may spread to the pelvis and eventually in the whole body.

Ovarian Cysts and Cancer: is most frequent tumor in the body. Every woman has a small cyst on the ovary, which may disappear spontaneously. The ovarian cyst causes distension of the abdomen and pressure on the organs such as the bladder or rectum. It should be removed by surgery without delay. Cancer may develop in the wall of ovarian cyst, may spread to other nearby organs causing obstruction of the bowel.

13

Problematic Deliveries

Surgical Delivery

Usually if the fetal head is stuck up higher up, a cesarean delivery is needed and surgery is required. Cesarean section should not be the last resort of the obstetrician after other methods of delivery have been attempted and have failed. Today, cesarean birth is a relatively safe, surgical operation in which the baby is born through the incision in the uterine and abdominal walls instead of through the vagina. An incision is made horizontally at the lower part of abdomen and the baby and placenta are removed through a cut in uterus and abdomen, closed by stitching. In an emergency delivery the baby is removed out by a long vertical cut. A cesarean birth may be indicated for the following reasons:

- **Pelvic disproportion**: A space problem resulting from a large baby or a small pelvic structure or a combination of the two.
- **Mal-presentation**: When the baby is situated unfavorably for a vaginal birth.
- **A prolonged labor**: Often, when the contractions are of poor quality or the dilation and descent are not progressing.
- **Fetal distress**: Due to changes in the fetal heart rate when the baby's oxygen supply has been reduced.
- **Prolapsed cord**: It occurs when the umbilical cord descends through the vagina before the baby is delivered resulting reduced oxygen supply.

- **Placenta previa**: When the placenta covers the cervix. As the cervix dilates, the placenta separates from the uterus depriving the fetus of oxygen.
- **Abruptio placenta**: When placenta prematurely separates from the uterine wall.
- **Maternal disease**: If the mother has toxemia, diabetes, high blood pressure, heart disease or other conditions, she or her baby may not be able to withstand the stress of labor and vaginal birth.
- **Repeat cesarean**: Sometimes, it is planned in advance because the original problem still exists or there may be risk of uterine rupture.
- **Heart disease in pregnancy**: Every attempt must be made top avoid cesarean section in these cases. A cardiac patient is not a suitable candidate for trial labor.

Complications: An incision is made in the middle line of the abdominal wall about six inches in length. Just before incising the uterus, it is desirable to give 0.25 mg. of methergine (strictly as advised by the doctor) intravenously directly into the uterine muscle to promote efficient uterine contraction and retraction. The suturing of the uterine incision immediately after the baby is delivered helps to control the hemorrhage. The placenta should be expressed by pressing the fundus and pushing out the placenta through incision in the utrine. Care should be taken before delivery of the head, to see that the incision is sufficiently long to allow the head to pass out comfortably.

Ectopic or tubal pregnancy

It is rare complication in which the fertilized ovum or embryo becomes blocked in its passage through the Fallopian tube. The embryo continues to grow as it normally would within the uterus. However, the space within the tube is too small to allow expansion, which may rupture causing a serious hemorrhage. Ectopic pregnancy is one of the leading causes of maternal death, with severe pain, abnormal vaginal bleeding and a palpable adnexal mass present in most of the patient in most of the patients. The factors increasing the risk of ectopic pregnancy include

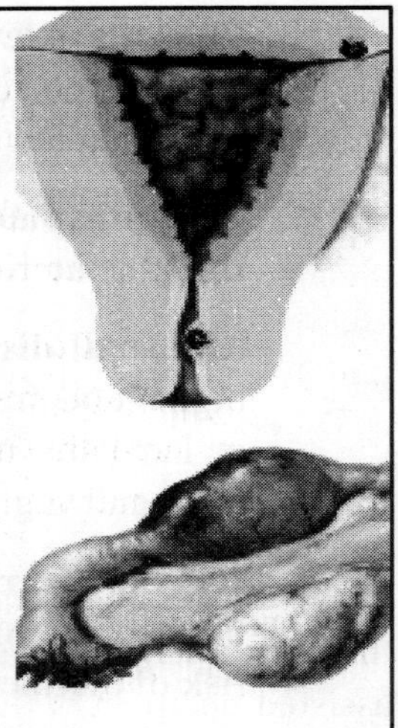

Ectopic Pregnancy

- Tubal abnormality resulting in delayed transit.
- Previous tubal pregnancy.
- Previous history of tubal reconstructive surgery.
- Intrauterine contraceptive devices and factors such as increased age and parity.

Induced delivery

In this delivery, labor is brought on or induced artificially by rupturing the membranes and letting out a little amniotic fluid, which stimulates labor pains. When the pains are too feeble or the deliver y is overdue, labor is induced through medicines to contract the uterus.

Premature delivery

The termination of pregnancy after the fetus become visible, such as capable of living independently is called premature birth. If the fetus is born dead, it is still- birth. Causes of abortion can also endanger the growth of the fetus resulting in a still- birth or premature delivery. Premature birth is usually the problem with the placenta to the faulty blood supply to the fetus, defective hormone production and effect of injurious toxins and chemicals through the blood to the fetus.

Precipitate labor

A precipitate labor lasts less than three hours. The latent phase of a precipitate labor passes unnoticed or so quickly and uneventfully that a pregnant miss the early signs of labor. If a hospital birth is planned, leave home hurriedly, trying to cope with strong, late labor contractions. If the pregnant is unaware that her labor is progressing rapidly and thinks she is in early labor with very painful contractions, she may feel unprepared, discouraged, experience feelings of loneliness a lack of direction, panic and unsure of her ability to handle labor. Take deep, slow and relaxing breaths. Have a vaginal examination before making any decision about anesthesia. When the second stage begins, lie on your side rather than using a gravity-assisted position, which will give your birth canal and perineum more time to stretch, decrease the likelihood of tearing and protect baby's head from being pressed through the vagina.

Prolonged labor

A labor that lasts longer than 24 hours is considered a prolonged labor. A labor with a long pre-labor or long latent phase can discourage, exhaust and emotionally drain the mother. On the other hand, a labor that slows or stops in the active phase or later may turn into a complication.

Emergency delivery

You may find it very disturbing if you had arranged your delivery in a hospital, and you have to change your plans to have baby at home. Don't feel panic, t is better to stay home than to attempt to rush to the hospital. The following suggestions will help you maintain control of an emergency situation and ensure the best possible outcome. The following are the signs of an imminent birth:

- Feeling of a strong urge to bear down.
- Baby's head or presenting part is visible at the vagina.
- Feeling of the baby coming out.

Call for someone to help you at home- your partner, a relative, a neighbor or a friend. You should immediately follow the following routine:

- Remove your clothes from the lower half of your body.
- Lie on the side or in a semi-sitting position in a warm, comfortable place, preferably on the bed with a waterproof sheet and clean towels or folded linen under her buttocks.
- Stay as relaxed as possible. Let the uterus do the work. Try not to push or bear down with the contractions. Keep tissues, clean towels and blanket nearby.
- During the birth, when baby's scalp is seen at the vagina, it will be wet and somewhat wrinkled, and it may be streaked with blood in places. The pressure of baby's head bulges the perineum and anus. With the contractions, more and more baby's head is visible. As baby's head descends, the expectant mother should expel the contents of her lower bowel. She must keep her thighs and pelvic floor relaxed. If the baby's head is delivered slowly, it lessens the risk of tearing the perineum.
- Once the head is fully emerged from the vagina, the partner or attendant should use the clean handkerchief to wipe away excess mucus from around the baby's nose and mouth. Wipe baby's face thoroughly. With the next contractions, the expectant mother delivers shoulders and rest of the body smoothly. Your partner or attendant can support the baby's wet and slippery body as it emerges.

Childbirth in the 8th month

Mostly an infant born in the 8th month doesn't survive. A 30 years old woman gave birth to a baby, which did not survive beyond 16 hours. Her second child too was born premature and died within 24 hours. Many natural salts including calcium are needed for the healthy growth of a child in the womb. If the diet of an expecting mother is deficient in these salts the fetus doesn't develop normally and the mother may suffer from weakness of muscles, which support the uterus and may have a miscarriage. Even if the delivery is normal, the child more often is sickly and too weak. Calcium is found in leafy vegetables and milk in abundant quantity and if an expecting mother takes a diet containing ample quantity of nutrients, she will deliver a healthy baby. She must seek advice of a doctor.

Pregnancy in women over 40 years old

Advanced age is considered to increase the likelihood of pregnancy and labor complications, especially in the first-time mother. The chances of complications include Down's syndrome in the baby, pre-eclampsia and poor labor pattern during pregnancy in women over 40. A healthy expectant mother over 40 can, however, enjoy the pregnancy.

Symptoms just before the delivery

Every expecting mother should be familiar with the symptoms as the time of confinement nears. At the time of childbirth, a woman requires lots of love, affection and confidence from her husband and family members to overcome the pain barrier. The following symptoms are observed just before a delivery:

- The sudden onset of labor pains is brought on by drop in the level of progesterone hormone.
- There is urge for frequent urination.
- The low position of the fetal head makes walking and sitting difficult.
- There is backache and tiredness in the limbs.
- Vaginal secretion increases; it may be blood- stained.
- The abdomen goes into regular, periodic tightness due to uterine contractions.

14

Venereal Diseases

Syphilis

A dangerous venereal disease caused by a little corkscrew-shaped germ. This tiny germ is transmitted from one person to another mainly through sexual contact. In a few cases syphilis is acquired through contaminated material and even through injections or blood transfusions, if the germs are present in the blood. If a mother is infected with syphilis, the germs may find their way into the child's' body before birth. Prominent signs and symptoms of disease in males is a painless sore on the penis lasting several weeks and in females there may be sore deep in the vagina. The early primary lesion is known as a Chancre. At first the germs are generally confined to these areas, and later they are carried to all parts of the body through the blood and spread causing mild rashes on the skin, which fade in a short time. Tumors or swellings may appear in various parts of the body and there may be severe inflammation and degeneration, which lead to headache, loss of memory, tremors of the lips, tongue, fingers, hands, change in the pupils of the eyes, loss of vision, vomiting acute abdominal pain lasting for hours or even days and developing large ulcers on the toes, heels and soles.

Pregnant women suffering from syphilis may pass on the disease to their unborn child in growing fetus resulting in serious conditions. Soon after the birth the bones of the child sometimes appear deformed, the liver and spleen enlarged, damage to the brain and central nervous system causing the birth of a mentally and physically retarded child. A syphilitic pregnant expectant mother runs the risk of recurrent abortions and stillbirths due to the infection, damage to placenta and the growing embryo. Here is a natural remedy to treat syphilis:

Ground in water a tablespoon of Hirankhuri booti (corchorus fascicularis) and few grains of pepper. Strain and take for two to three weeks. The patient should take a salt-free diet and avoid taking bitter, sour and pungent substances.

Gonorrhea

Persistent pus discharge from vagina, inflammation of entire genital passage, burning and discomfort are symptoms of Gonorrhea - a fatal venereal disease usually transmitted by sexual contact caused by a tiny bean-shaped germ called a 'gonococcus'. The disease may also be contracted from contaminated hands, instruments, clothing, toilet seats, and even bath water. Burning on urination, urge to frequent urination, a profuse, greenish-yellow discharge, red and swollen end of the penis in males and hot, swollen opening to the vagina along with thick yellow discharge are some of the symptoms of this disease. Adult men and women carry gonorrhea germs transmitted during sexual intercourse. If a mother happens to be infected with gonorrhea, there is great danger of newborn infant contracting the disease at the time of birth. In the males the prostate gland becomes infected resulting in slow urination. In females the Fallopian tubes get closed as a result of formation of abscess and the inflammation in the pelvis. The following treatments cure gonorrhea.

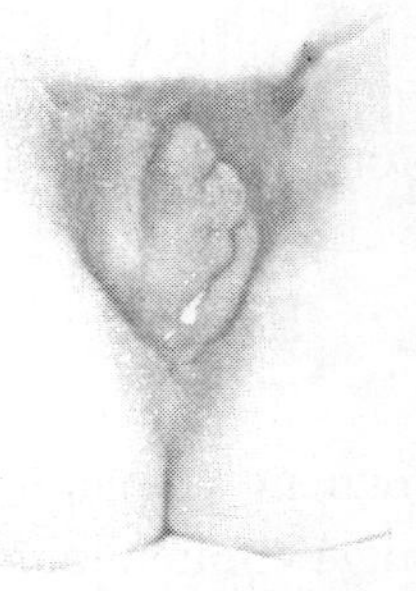

Gonorrhea

Penicillin or Terramycin is the best drugs recommended for the treatment of this fatal disease (strictly under the guidance of an expert doctor as there may be a reaction due to these drugs). A Hip Bath in hot water is useful. Urethra should be flushed with a solution of potassium permanganate (1:3000) with the help of a syringe to be kept in urethra for five minutes. The patient should avoid constipation. Sex should be strictly forbidden.

Genital herpes

Herpes simplex virus produces infection generally passed on through sexual contact. Appearance of blisters on genital areas, thighs, buttocks, fever, body ache, weakness, thick vaginal discharge, irritation, urinary burning and enlarged lymph nodes are some of the symptoms of this disease. Different sized vesicles and reddish ulcers appear in the vulvae region. Women who practice rectal sex also develop the lesions in the area around the anus and higher up in the rectum. This disease is treated by the application of anti-viral cream or a lotion. Use condoms during sexual intercourse. Take bath in warm water. Worry, depression and lack of sleep are biggest enemies during the attack of this disease. Soothe the affected skin with essential oil (diluted in a base oil) of lemon, geranium, chamomile or lavender. The oil should be gently rubbed on to the rash.

Fungus infection

Occasionally, the female genital organs of a pregnant woman get infected with fungus because of the increased sugar content in the blood. Women suffering from diabetes are more likely to have fungus infections resulting in intense itching around the genital area and a thick discharge from the vagina. Take a warm vinegar douche once or twice a day in consultation with your doctor.

Leucorrhoea (Vaginal discharge)

The secretion from the uterus and upper portion of the vagina flowing down and reabsorbed in the lower part of the vagina is a normal phenomena in a woman. The presence of infection in any of these tissues usually causes a whitish or pale discharge sometime accompanied by pus is called leucorrhoea. Pelvic congestion, endocrine disturbances, lacerations, injuries, perhaps atrophy of the vaginal tissues, an irritation of the labia (external genital organs in young girls), soiled undergarments, dirt, intestinal worms and masturbation are some of the causes of this disease. Excess secretion is common when the girl reaches puberty due to over activity in sex glands and organs. Sometimes, young women are having slight discharge at the time of ovulation, which is not abnormal nor indicate the presence of any disease.

A profuse, yellowish discharge associated with burning and intense itching while urinating may be due to infectious disease gonorrhea. A thin, watery discharge may be due to the presence of cancer in the uterus or cervix. A creamy, slightly blood stained discharge may be due to some severe infection. From the early pregnancy period to mid forties, infections may sometimes follow the birth of a child because of the cervix been damaged during delivery of the baby. Unless properly treated, infection may spread to other areas of the genital tract, even leading to cancer. A Pap smear, blood test and the skin test should always be done if there is a yellowish discharge. Strong antibiotic treatment, however, subside infection. Take a regular vinegar douche. Mix two tablespoons of vinegar to ½ liter warm water. After douching, a vaginal suppository or table should be inserted in the vagina. In case of severe itching, triple sulphonamide cream may be applied inside the genital organ (as prescribed by a doctor) to control infection. Cream containing the hormone estrogen when applied locally will benefit. In case of female infection the husband should be carefully examined and treated. A leucorrhoea patient should undertake regular exercise. Late nights and sexual intercourse are taboo during the course of disease. Avoid fried. Spicy foods and pickles.

Excessive bleeding

Menstrual bleeding occurs in all women from adolescence till the menopausal change of life. Women, sometimes also have slight signs of blood on the day of ovulation, which is normal. Heavy vaginal bleeding during the childbearing age may be due to the miscarriage of abortion, ectopic pregnancy and malignant tumors of the uterus or cervix. Women with irregular or very heavy bleeding should have a Pap test done at least every six months. Heavy bleeding may also be due to fibroid tumors and polyps in the uterus. In such cases either the tumor or perhaps the entire uterus have be removed. Various other conditions, such as blood diseases, heart failure, alcoholism, cirrhosis of the liver, vitamin B deficiencies, and abnormality in either thyroid or pituitary, or adrenal glands may result in heavy bleeding. Heavy bleeding following abortion usually requires a surgical operation to clean uterus whereas bleeding arising from tumors of the uterus and other pelvic organs is controlled by surgery.

If the woman is in mid-pregnancy and suddenly begins to hemorrhage, she should be rushed to hospital at once otherwise it may be too late to save the baby as well as mother's life. All the products of conception should be expelled from the uterus, otherwise bleeding may not cease and there is danger of serious infection in the uterus.

Candida (white vaginal thrush)

Females during reproductive age sometimes suffer from candida. Factors like the state of pregnancy, diabetes, administration of antibiotics and steroids and use of contraceptive pills cause this disorder, which produces white vaginal discharge with intense irritation and burning sensation. To treat affected area, apply anti-fungal cream recommended for both men and women to eliminate the fungus and prevent re-infection from the sex partner. In case of females, doctors generally recommend tablets inserted intra-vaginally. Thrush is another infection of candida usually develops in the gastro-intestinal tract. Whitish curd-like deposits appear on the tongue. The thrush infection of vagina is known as vulva vaginitis, which cause itching, redness and discharge. The vaginal infection can be transmitted to the male partner and vice versa. Symptoms of vaginitis include:

1. Pain, redness and itching into the vagina and vulva.
2. Severe pain when urinating and involved in sexual intercourse.
3. Foul smelling white or blood-streaked discharge.
4. Pelvic inflammation resulting in infertility.

The following measures are taken for the treatment of vaginitis (strictly as prescribed by your doctor):

- Avoid wearing nylon panties, tight jeans and a moist environment around genital area.
- Avoid sugar, refined carbohydrates and alcohol, which turn into glucose in the body.
- Eat 100 gm of unsweetened yogurt daily.
- Garlic is antibacterial, anti-fungal that fights both bacterial vaginitis and candidiasis. Take one capsule once or twice a day.
- Insert a 600 mg capsule of boric acid powder into vagina twice a day for a week. To prevent recurrence insert one capsule daily at bed time for four days during menstrual period. Do not insert capsule in case of pregnancy.
- Insert a vitamin E capsule into the vagina once or twice a day for seven days, which is soothing to vaginal tissue, decreases irritation, redness, swelling and congestion.
- Ayurvedic herb 'triphla' helps remove toxins from the body and helps in treating a yeast infection. Soak ½ teaspoon of dried herb in 1 cup of hot water for five minutes. Drink the liquid at night before sleep. Douching, too, dries the vagina.

Common conditions of genitalia

Scabies, warts, herpes, candidiasis, phimosis and AIDS virus are some of common conditions of Genitalia.

Lesions of scabies: may be seen on male genitals with intense itching. These lesions are observed as papules on the prepuce, glans, shaft of penis and scrotum in male organs. Female genitalia are rarely involved.

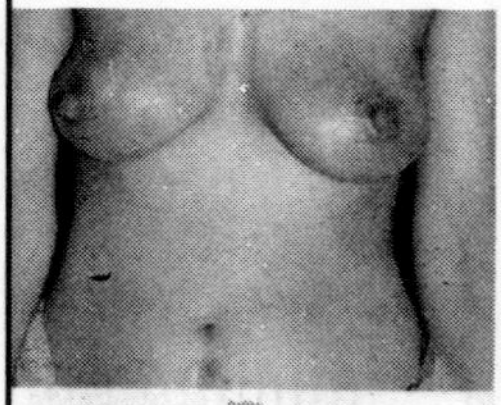
Scabies on Female Body

Surface warts: also do occur on genitalia. Genital warts are usually transmitted by sexual contact or through infection from the hands and nail, as such both the partners should keep hands clean when having sex. Warts can occur in both sexes and are usually located on the moist surface of genitalia. Initially, they appear as minute reddish swellings growing in groups of lesions. The genital warts should be treated with the consultation of a good doctor.

Remedies to genital herpes: are caused by a virus, in which groups of little blisters appear on the genital area, thighs and buttocks. The following natural remedies for genital herpes are recommended:

- Vitamins and minerals: A herpes outbreak is a sign that your body is under stress and needs more nutrients. The following nutrient program may help reduce the stress, shorten the herpes attack and reduce its severity:

Vitamin A: Daily dose of 20,000 international units (IU) twice for a week.

Vitamin B Complex: Daily dose 50 mg for a month.

Vitamin C: Daily dose 500 to 1000 mg three times a day for one to two weeks.

Vitamin E: 400 IU twice a day for two weeks.

Zinc: 10 mg twice a day for a week.

Calcium/Magnesium: 500 mg of calcium and 250 mg of magnesium twice a day for a month.

Selenium: 200 micrograms daily for two weeks.

- Drink water as much as you can, which helps flush toxins

out of the body that weaken immune system and allow the virus to reactivate.

- Soothe group of little blisters appearing on genital area with essential oils (diluted in a base oil) of lemon, geranium, chamomile or lavender.
- Common warts are treated by electro-cautery, which excises the warts with electric current.

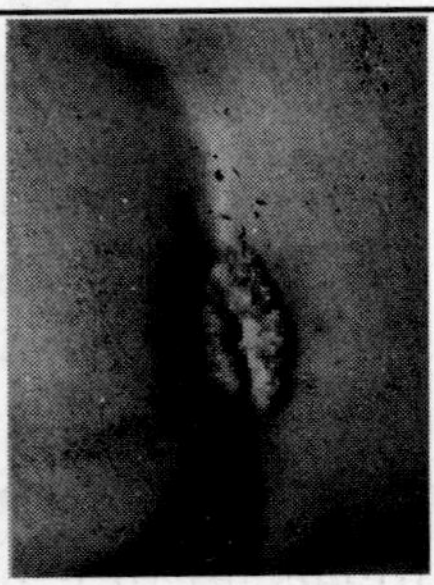

Peri-Anal Warts

Remedies to cure warts: Warts should be diagnosed accurately and treated early rather than waiting until they spread and enlarge and are more difficult to eliminate. Genital warts can be sexually transmitted and may be a risk factor for cervical cancer in women. The following natural remedies are suggested:

- Garlic oil is a traditional remedy for warts. Swab the oil on the wart or on a bandage applied to the wart.
- Remove warts with cryosurgery or freezing with liquid nitrogen or carbon snow.

Remedies for treating scabies: Scabies is a contagious disease caused by a mite, which lays eggs in burrows in the skin. The disease spreads through contact with infected individual. The commonly affected parts of the body are finger webs, wrist, arms, buttocks, lower abdomen, thighs, breast-folds, female genital area and penis (in men). There is severe itching on the affected area at night and sometimes thin, slimy fluid oozes out of the scratched surface and scabs. To treat scabby following remedies are advised:

- Boil leaves of oleander (Karbir) till charred in 250 ml mustard oil and massage the affected skin.
- Mix juices of lemon and jasmine in equal quantity and rub on the itching skin.
- Grind poppy seeds in water. Mix to it lime juice. Massage affected skin with the paste.

15

Skin Diseases Associated With Pregnancy

In a study conducted on pregnant women most of them were found to have any lesion involving the skin. The following are the more important physiological changes, which affect the skin of the pregnant woman as described below:

Pigmentation

Present in about 75% of all pregnant women by the last trimester. It usually regresses after delivery, but it may persist for varying periods of time and occasionally until the menopause. The commonest and most characteristic site for pigmentation is the face and the forehead where it is known as 'Chloasma'. The cause of pregnancy pigmentation is due to increased production of progesterone, which directly affects the melanocytes. Other pigmentary changes occurring during pregnancy are the following:

- Hyper-pigmentation of pigmented areas especially of the vulva and labia, areola, nipples and umbilicus.
- Pigmentation of linea alba usually developing in the 3rd month of pregnancy.
- The linea nigra fusca – pigmentation running from the mons to the umbilicus.
- Pigment marks on and around the areola on breasts.

Alteration in the growth of hair (hypertrichosis)

Excess growth of hair on the face, which usually disappears after delivery but reappear in subsequent pregnancies.

Striae Gravidarum

Almost 75% women usually suffer from this disorder by the 6th month of pregnancy, which appear as thin, clear-cut lines of atrophy in parallel or in curves on abdomen, breasts, flanks, lumbar and sacral regions, hips and inner side of thighs. The lines become less conspicuous with the passage of time after delivery.

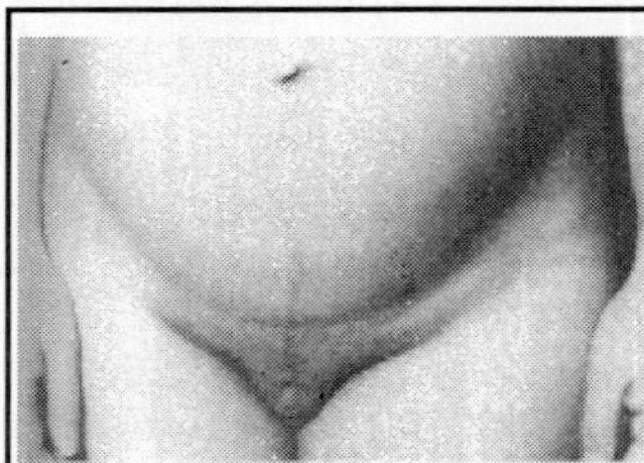

Lines running from cubus

Erythema of palms

Present as mottled erythema distributed on entire surface of the palm, which increases with the advance of pregnancy. Erythema is found to be present in 60% of fair complexioned women and 40% of dark complexioned women. It fades in 90% of cas3s within 6 to 8 weeks after delivery.

Multiple spider naevi

Bright red lesions usually appear between second and fifth month of pregnancy and slowly increase in size mainly on the face, neck, upper arms and chest. About 75% of the lesions disappear completely within two months of delivery and sometimes remain un-curable even for years. The cause of spider naevi is due to hormonal reasons.

Molluscum fibroma gravidarum

These contagious lesions also caused by virus due to epidermal hyperplasia and consist of a core of connective tissues without any elastic tissue covered by epidermis. They appear during second half of pregnancy on the front, sides, nape of the neck, in the axillae, on the breast and upper chest.

Skin diseases related to pregnancy

These include pruigo gestationis, herpes gestationis, impeligo herpetiformus, papular dermatitis of pregnancy, lesions of prurigo, macules, papules, excoriations, lichenification, urticarial eruptions, eczematous eruptions, erythemas and scabies. Most of these eruptions develop in late pregnancy. Irritation and rashes disappear in 7 to 14 days with proper medication prescribed by the doctor.

Herpes gestationis

Lesions develop in first pregnancy or during the successive pregnancies due to hormonal changes in which lesions develop during the second trimester of pregnancy and usually itching and burning between the age 30 to 35 years. It starts clearing within 30 days after the pregnancy. Recurrences occur on the resumption of menstruation and in rare occasions the disease has made first appearance in the puerperium. The patches may become pustular or haemorrhagia and the rashes spread. Eventually the whole body may be involved. The lesions regress and heal leaving behind pigmentation. Constitutional symptom such as pyrexia, rigors, constipation, vomiting and proteinuria accompanies the eruption.

Impetigo herpetiformis

An inflammatory condition of the skin accompanied by severe constitutional disturbance with pyrexia, rigors, vomiting and delirium is conspicuous, which cannot be identified by the primary lesions, pustule in groups containing pus. The eruption having yellow crust spreads, oozes and resembles eczema. Most of the children born of mother suffering from this disease die soon after the birth.

Papular dermatitis of pregnancy

The symptoms include intense itching lesions widely scattered over the trunk, arms, legs, face and scalp throughout the pregnancy. The condition is associated with a high fetal morality. Consult a doctor for treatment.

Intertrigo (intertriginous dermatitis)

An highly inflammatory reaction of the epidermis, which occur in the region of the body folds or area on the skin surfaces in close contact. Such areas include the axillary folds, inguinal folds, inter-gluteal cleft and inter-digital cleft of toes. The causes of this disease are friction, sweating and heat, which lead inevitably to reddening, scales, soreness and irritation and maceration of the epidermis of skin followed by infection, erosions and fissures with skin organism, fungi or yeasts especially candida albicans. The diagnosis of this skin disorder during pregnancy must be made from flexural psoriasis, seborrhoeic dermatitis, eczema, fungal infection and monilial infection. The treatment includes soothing the inflammation, keeping affected skin clean with soap and water, sitz baths or foot baths of potassium permanganate solution for minimum 10 minutes or wet dressings of potassium permanganate, application of steroid lotions or creams and fungicidal ointment, control over obesity, diabetes and glycosuria.

Psoriasis

The skin disease is common during pregnancy on limbs and trunk usually due to friction, moisture and overweight. To cure psoriasis, warm or potassium permanganate baths are suggested followed by application of steroid lotion or cream. If untreated, it leads to the risk of irritant dermatitis or sensitization.

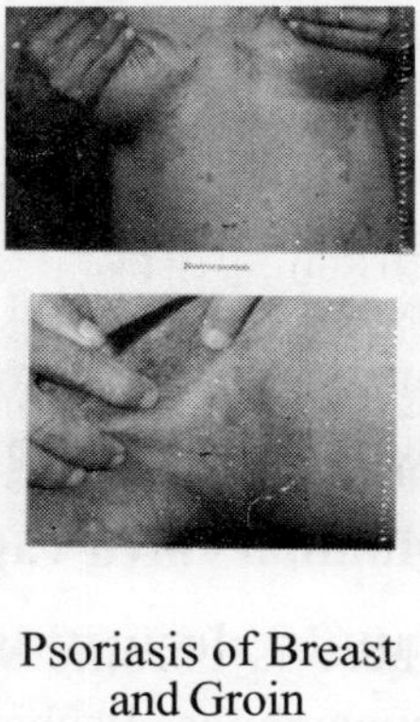

Psoriasis of Breast and Groin

Eczema and scabies

The areola and the nipple are common sites

for eczema on the body of a pregnant woman having eczematous lesions on the breasts, wrists, anterior and posterior axillary folds usually appearing on skin creases.

Condyloma Acuminate

When warts start oozing, growing rapidly in pregnant women with offensive odor generally affecting external genitalia, pre-anal region and perineum. This contagious virus disease of the skin spreads in moist medium and become very proliferative in the presence of vaginal discharges due to presence of venereal diseases (especially gonorrhea) or other infections. To have a curb over disease scrupulous cleanliness of affected area is essential and all vaginal discharges should be investigated.

Pityriasis versicolor

It is a fungus skin disease in pregnant women generally characterized by round macules. The color of lesions varies from light to deep brown giving an appearance of hyper-pigmentation accompanied by scales. It is difficult to cure this disease during pregnancy. To treat the disorder wash the affected areas thoroughly having daily hot bath, application of a 10% solution of sodium thiosulphate with a brush or applying ointment containing sulphur and salicylic acid.

Candidiasis (cutaneous moniliasis)

Nearly 25% of pregnant women suffer from this disease in the vaginal area and attribute to the increased amount of glycogen present in the vaginal cells. Candidiasis is classified into three groups: cutaneous and mucosal thrush, secondary eruptions due to yeasts and monilial granulomata.

Monilial vulvo-vaginitis

There is chronic vaginal discharge in this disorder. Heavy leucorrhoea discharge during pregnancy causes fungus. The symptoms include pruritus vulvae and soreness of introitus, odema, excoriation and lichenification of the labia and perineal region, congestion and reddening of the vaginal mucosa, white patches accompanied by fungus on the labia and vaginal wall. Consult a doctor immediately. The remedial measures include daily sitz bath in the solution of potassium permanganate solution, insertion of nystatin pessaries into the vagina at night and in the morning. For 2 to 4 weeks in consultation with your doctor and application of nystatin ointment or powder (as recommended by the doctor).

Trichomoniasis

Infection is the common cause of vaginal discharge and vulvo-vaginitis occurring in pregnant and non-pregnant women; also found during the post-menopausal periods in virgins, which may be transmitted to the male during intercourse giving rise to urethritis, palano-posthitis and chronic prostatitis. The main symptoms of this disease are pruritus vulvae, odema and redness of vulva with frothy vaginal discharge. To clear infection, oral therapy and insertion of pessaries have shown 80% curative effects. If repeated relapses occur in married women, it is advisable to treat the husband also.

Malignant melanoma

High malignant, dangerous pigmented flat, brown moles on the head, neck, lower limbs and trunk appear. The irritating lesions rapidly increase in size developing dark pigmentation, ooze watery discharge on outer zone. The lesions are diagnosed by pigmented basal cell and squamous epithelioma, pigmented papilloma, seborrhoeic wart, haemangioma pigmented naevi and solar keratosis. Patients already suffering from malignant melanoma are warned that pregnancy carries the risk of activation and dissemination of any metastasis.

Pruritus in pregnancy

Common skin disorder during 2nd and 3rd trimester of pregnancy, which interferes with sleep and exhaust the patient mentally and physically, localized to the vulva or peri-anal regions often associated with pain, itching, striae gravidarum, urticaria, scabies and varicosities of the vulva. The causes of generalized pruritus include dermatoses related to pregnancy, metabolic disorders (such as diabetes, jaundice and uraemia), leukemia (blood dyscrasiois), skin diseases (eczema, dermatitis, scabies, herpetiformis and herpes gestationis), malignant abdominal and pelvic diseases, lack of personal cleanliness, bacterial infection of inguinal folds, excessive vaginal discharge, pediculosis pubis, use of contraceptive pessaries and creams, contact dermatitis due to due to sanitary pads and nylon underclothes. To treat the disorder, remove the cause, if possible. Apply corticosteroid creams or lotions in consultation with the doctor. Tepid baths are helpful to treat this disorder.

16

Stages of Labor

Labor is divided into four stages as below:

- First Stage-the Dilating stage: During which the cervix opens completely.
- Second Stage-the Expulsion stage: Also called actual birth, which begins when the cervix is fully dilated and ends when the baby is born.
- Third Stage-the Placental stage: Begins with the birth of the baby and ends with the delivery of the placenta.
- Fourth Stage-the Recovery stage: Which begins after the placenta is born and ends one to several hours later when the mother's condition stabilizes.

Dilation and signs of labor

When the gestation period is over, the baby is about to be delivered, the mother starts getting severe labor pains. Following types of women feel less pain during delivery:

- Accustomed to domestic work.
- Do regular morning and evening walk.
- Do regular exercise
- Have sound health and well-developed pelvis.

Dilation refers to the opening of the cervix. It is usual for the cervix to dilate slightly before the onset of labor. The dilation is estimated during a vaginal examination and is measured in centimeters. When the cervix is opened only a fingertip, it is one centimeter dilated, at the halfway point, it is four to five centimeters and when fully dilated, it is eight to ten centimeters dilated. The prominent signs of labor are the following:

- Backache that come and go accompanied by uneasiness and restlessness.
- Frequent soft bowel movements often mistaken for an intestinal upset. Diarrhea-like symptoms on or near your due date may be a subtle sign of early labor.
- Passage of a thickened mucus plug tinged with blood from the rupture blood vessels in the cervix, which can appear days before any other sign of labor.
- Contractions of uterus become longer, stronger and closer together as labor advances. Contractions usually become painful near the delivery period. Uterine contractions shorten the muscle fibers in the body of the uterus, pull open the cervix and push the fetus down and out of the uterus.
- Rupture of the membranes or breaking of the bag of waters begins labor usually immediately or within 24 hours. When the membranes break, followed by a gush of amniotic fluid (or a slow, uncontrollable leak of fluid may feel like urination). When rupture of membrane occurs and labor doesn't begin the risk of infection increases as time passes. Seek medical advise and note the time, color, odor and amount of fluid. Do not insert anything into your vagina to control the flow. Avoid inserting fingers, having intercourse and taking a tub bath. That can increase the possibility of infection.

Pain in childbirth

There are several factors as below:

- Insufficient supply of oxygen to uterine muscles. The pain is more intense if the interval between contractions is short.
- Stretching of the cervix.
- Pressure by the baby on the nerves near the cervix and vagina.
- Tension on and stretching of the supporting ligaments of the uterus and surrounding structures during structures.
- Pressure on the urethra, bladder and rectum.
- Distention of the pelvic floor muscles.
- Fear and anxiety, which release excessive stress hormones.

Pelvic examination before labor

The objects are twofold- to investigate the condition of the pelvic organs and to estimate the size and shape of the pelvic canal. It is necessary to measure the pelvis by your doctor by means of a bimanual examination. The diagnosis of pregnancy is confirmed and the presence or absence of pelvic swellings such as uterine fibroids or ovarian cysts can be determined. If the fundus (top of the uterus) can be palpated abdominally there is no need to carry out the pelvic examination at the first visit and can be postponed until need arises. There are three methods of pelvic examination as below:

1. External Examination: The measurements are made with a pair of calipers to find out any deformity to be recognized at once.
2. Internal Examination: Interspinous diameter is measured with hands. The two, anterior-superior spines are located, where fingers are placed on their outer lips and the

measurement read off. Normally it is generally 24 –25 cm. in average pregnant. The Intercristal diameter is also measured round the iliac cresta. This measurement is normally 26-27 cm.

3. By X-rays: The size of the pelvis and the fetal head can be assessed by X-ray. This process is known as Radiographic Pelvimetry.

Preparations before delivery

The following things should be kept ready before delivery:

- A hard bed to avoid excess labor pains.
- Oily cloth for spreading on the bed.
- Two rolls of sterilized cotton wool.
- Few napkins duly rinsed in carbolic lotion and dried.
- Two basins, each for membranes and waste cotton.
- Enema pot, boric acid and anti-septic lotion.
- Four binders of size 36" long and 16" broad for stomach required immediately after the delivery.
- Four loin clothes to manage vagina.

Just before and after delivery

Labor is divided into three stages as described below. The first stage lasts about 12-15 hours, the second stage about two hours and the third stage takes 20 minutes to half an hour. In the patients belonging to working class, the average time is considerably shorter. The first stage occupies 8-10 hours, the second stage one hour or less and the third stage 20 minutes to half an hour. These are average figures and labor class women usually complete their labor in a much shorter time.

Stage of dilation (The first stage of labor)

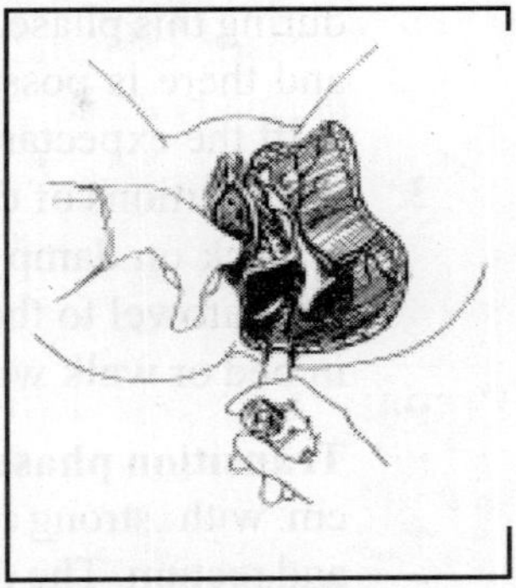

Start from the onset of true pains to the full dilation of the cervix. The occurrence includes periodic pain due to contraction of the uterus and therefore synchronous with a hardening of that organ, which can be felt by hands are placed on abdomen. There is continuous discharge from vagina (cervical mucosa), also known as 'show'. As the pain becomes more frequent and severe, the patient begins to cry out. And feels relief by sitting bent forward. A gentle massage on the back from shoulder to lower back is also helpful for the patient to relieve tension. It takes 12 to 15 hours to complete the first stage. At the end of it there is usually a sudden gush of fluid indicating that the fetal membranes have ruptured.

Birth guide during 1st stage

There are three phases in this stage such as lateral stage, active stage and transition stage as per the following detail:

- **Lateral phase**: The cervix dilation occurs from 1 to 4 cm. The breathing pattern should remain slow. Sometimes, there is bloody show during this stage. The contractions become longer, stronger and more frequent with small chance of rupture of membranes. The delivering woman may have backache and loose bowel movements. She should frequently empty bladder (every hour) and eat and drink sensibly according to desire. She must bathe or shower and feel relaxed as far as possible. It is suggested to call doctor or midwife. The husband/partner should help pass the time with walking, talking, music, TV and back rub.

- **Active phase**: The cervix dilation ranges from 5 to 7 cm. during this phase when contractions become more intense and there is possibility of rupture of membranes. Better shift the expectant mother to the nursing home. She must use positions of comfort, drink liquids, chew on ice chips or suck on damp cloth, apply cool cloth to her forehead, warm towel to the abdomen, have ice or liquid and move in bed or walk with the help of her husband or partner.
- **Transition phase**: The cervix dilation varies from 8 to 10 cm. with strong contractions and heavy pressure on vagina and rectum. The delivering woman feels nausea, vomiting (or vomiting sensation), drowsiness, hiccups, cold feet uncontrollable shaking and frequent leg cramps. There is always possibility of rupture of membranes. The expectant mother feels restless, irritable, forgetful, fearful, often control urge to push and have difficulty with breathing. She should not be left alone. Back rubbing provides her comfort.

Stage of expulsion (The second stage of labor)

This is a stage of expulsion and extends from the complete dilation of the cervix to the expulsion of the child. The pains often stop for few minutes after the rupture and then begin again with greater frequency, which gradually become more expulsive or 'down bearing' in character. The patient usually braces herself by holding on to some solid object or pressing her feet against the foot of the bed. The diaphragm is thus fixed and the intra-abdominal pressure brought to bear on the expulsion of the child. The patient perspires freely. The effect of these pains is to drive the head through the cavity of the pelvis. It presses upon the rectum and on the perineum, which begins to bulge a little during the pains. The vulva also begins to gape more. Gradually, the pains become longer and more frequent, the head recede a little, but with each succeeding pain it is driven a little farther down. The perineum bulges more and more, the vulva too gapes more and more and the scalp of the baby is seen when the head is forced down during a pain. Larger and larger area of the head comes to lie in the vulva opening during successive pains. The opening becomes transformed from a slightly gaping slit to an oval and ultimately an almost circular opening. The perineum meantime has been so pressed that it becomes stretched out and thinned. After the head is born, there is a short pause during which the face of the child becomes congested. After the head, the shoulders, the trunk and lower limbs are pushed out, followed by a gush of the remainder of the liquor amnii. After the end of the second stage the retracted uterus may be felt as a firm tumor extending up to just below the umbilicus.

Birth guide during 2nd stage

The expectant mother have possible full contractions in this stage when urge to push becomes stronger due to pressure of stretching vagina and physical signs of birth of baby's head, then body. She must relax perineum, buttocks, legs and change position for comfort and as necessary. Remove the clothing from the lower half of the body. Lie on the side or in semi-sitting position in a warm comfortable place with clean towels or folded linen under the buttocks. A waterproof sheet will protect the mattress. Stay as relaxed as possible.

Stage of Delivery (The third stage of labor)

This is stage of delivery of child and extends from the birth of the child to the birth of the placenta. There is usually a short cessation of pains with a corresponding relief to the patient. Ultimately, the uterus begins to contract again, and may be felt by the hand to grow more hard and solid. Sometimes, there are little gushes of blood during the pains, indicating the separation of the placenta. Many times there is no bleeding. In the end, the placenta is expelled out by strong pain in the vagina. The third stage may take a few minutes to an hour or even more. The average time is about 20 minutes.

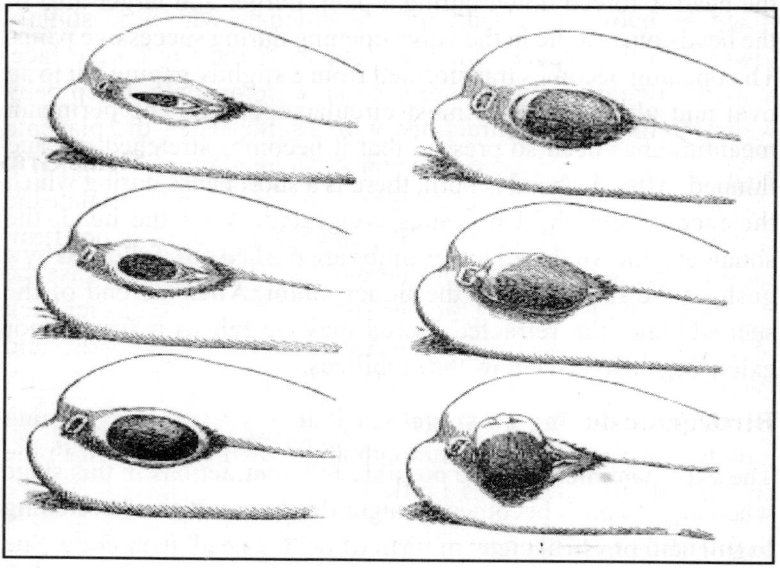

Birth guide during 3rd stage

The breathing pattern should be slow or accelerated breathing. She may try to push to expel placenta. There are mild to moderate contractions and uncontrollable shaking during this period. Excitement, fatigue and engrossment with baby are possible emotional signs an expectant mother may experience. The mother should push placenta out as directed and hold baby skin to skin. When you first see the baby's scalp at the vagina, it will be wet and wrinkled and may be streaked with blood. Pressure of the baby's head bulges perineum and anus. If the head is delivered slowly, it lessens the risk of tearing the perineum. Keep thighs and pelvic floor relaxed as the head emerges from the vagina. Once the head has fully emerged, the attendant should use the clean handkerchief to wipe away excess mucus from around the baby's nose and mouth. If the cord is around the baby's neck, the attendant should lift it gently over the baby's head.

Usually the baby begins breathing and crying immediately.

Place the baby on the side on bare abdomen with head slightly lower than the body to drain any mucus remaining on the face. Wipe away any mucus and dry the baby completely. Keep baby warm. Remember, contractions will resume when the placenta separates from the uterine wall and slide down into the vagina. A mother can start breastfeeding right away, which will stimulate the uterus to contract and reduce bleeding. If the uterus is not firm, massage the fundus (top of the uterus) until it contracts. In case the newly born baby does not breathe spontaneously, rub his/her back or chest briskly but gently. If not respond within 30 seconds, hold baby's feet together and smack the soles sharply. If still doesn't respond then mouth to mouth resuscitation is required by placing mouth over baby's nose and mouth and blowing gently air in the cheeks until the chest rises a little.

Separation of placenta

The resumption of pains after the birth of child indicates still further contraction and retraction of the upper segment. This brings about such a disproportion between the placental site and the placenta when the attachments between the two are torn through. The placental site may be reduced in area 4-1/2 by 4 inches (11 by 10 cm.) without separation taking place.

There are two methods of expulsion of placenta:

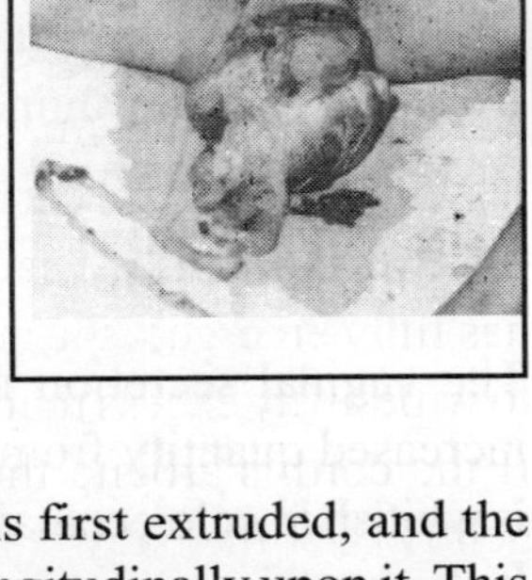

- **Schultze's method:** In which the placenta is expelled like an inverted umbrella when the fetal surface comes first and the membrane trailing behind.
- **Dubcan's mechanism:** Its also known as Matthews Duncan. In it the lower edge of the placenta is first extruded, and the whole organ slides down folded longitudinally upon it. This method is more common.

4th stage (Recovery)

First hours after birth is known as the 4th stage in which the delivered mother must breathe slowly. This is the stage when she feels shaking, have after-pains (painful uterine contractions), perineal discomforts, fatigue, exhaustion, empty feeling, difficulty while urination, hunger and nausea. She has desire to see and hold baby. Rest and relaxation are important factors at this stage. She must drink or eat, urinate (sitting up helps), massage fundus and apply ice pack to perineum to decrease discomfort and swelling.

How to control hemorrhage?

As the placenta is separated from the wall of the uterus, the blood vessels passing from the one to the other are torn across, and many of the large sinuses in the uterine wall thus laid open. Bleeding from these is, however, prevented by the very retraction of the uterus, which causes the separation. If owing to exhaustion of the uterus, retraction fails to occur after the separation of the placenta, then free and alarming bleeding may take place – known as postpartum hemorrhage.

Some bleeding will occur after labor and delivery. If there is blood loss more than two cups, the mother may be hemorrhaging characterizing by a steady flow of blood and symptoms of shock with rapid pulse, paleness, trembling, cold and sweating. On suspecting hemorrhage firmly massage the uterus through the abdominal wall until it contracts. If the bleeding appears to ooze from tears at the vaginal opening, pad the perineum with an ice pack and towels.

Vaginal secretion

The vaginal secretion in a healthy pregnancy differs only in its increased quantity from that of a healthy non-pregnant woman. It is whitish in color, containing epithelial cells, leucocytes and mucus. It also contains numerous large 'vaginal bacilli'. It has been observed that the acidity of the vaginal secretion is inimical to the life of other organism than the 'vaginal bacillus', followed by the appearance of organism in the vagina. Thus during the puerperium the lochia (discharge from the uterus after labor) is alkaline, which contain many organisms, mostly saprophytic are found.

Method of cleaning genitals after labor

Nature follows the principles of antisepsis in labor. The birth canal can be divided into three parts:

- The vulva (the entrance to vagina): This area swarms with organism of various sorts. It may therefore be designated the Septic tract.
- The vagina: The portion containing the vaginal bacilli with their acid secretion, a few fungi, and some leucocytes. This is Antiseptic tract.
- The cavity of the uterus: Separated by the plug of mucus from the vagina, is entirely devoid of any form of organism. It is therefore the Aseptic tract.

Wherever possible the patient should have a complete bath at the very commencement of labor, and the nurse should see that the rectum and bladder are emptied. It is usually suggested that the patient should be given an enema in every case, irrespective of whether the bowels have acted naturally or not, unless the patient is in strong labor when the nurse arrives. The nurse should then pay special attention to the genitals. The hair should be shaved. Before a vaginal examination is made the vulva is swabbed with a antiseptic solution. The labia minora must be separated and wiped with pledget of wool soaked in an antiseptic solution. The pledget must always be drawn from being backwards to prevent carrying forward any septic matter from near the anus. No pledget must be used for more than one wipe.

Puerperal infection

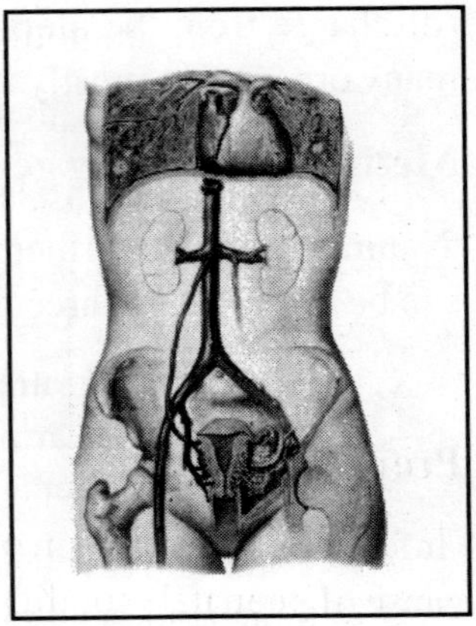

The term puerperal infection can be used to describe any infection during or after labor, it generally applies to infection of the uterus and surrounding tissues after delivery. This can vary from mild to life threatening in severity. Some of the most severe infections may appear within hours of the delivery and are often opportunistic and non-associated with reliable risk factors. Vigilance and aggressive diagnosis and treatment are required. The puerperal infection causes due to colonization and infection of the tissues of uterus, peritoneum or surrounding organs. Abscesses usually contain both aerobic and anaerobic bacteria. Nearly 50% of the ascending uterine infections involve harmful bacteria due to lack of cleanliness. The risk factors of this infection includes a Cesarean delivery, invasive procedure during labor, prolonged rupture of the membranes, prolonged labor, multiple examinations, retained placental fragments, urinary catheter, intravenous line(s), low socioeconomic status and chronic diseases including diabetes.

The signs and symptoms of the infection are fever and tachycardia often developing rapidly after delivery, uterine tenderness, sign of septic or cardiovascular shock, hypertension, anxiety, disorientation, prostration, impaired renal function, hemolysis or hemoconcentration. The infection can be diagnosed by the following symptoms:

- Urinary tract infection with the presence of large numbers of white blood cells.
- Wound infection.

- Infection in intravenous line or site and contaminated fluids.
- Disturbed abscess.
- Septic thrombophlebitis, necrotizing fasciitis, transfusion reaction, amniotic fluid or pulmonary embolism.
- Cardiogenic shock and toxic shock syndrome.
- Mastitis and afelectasis.
- Possible associated conditions such as septic shock, adult respiratory distress syndrome, acute renal failure and disseminated intra-vascular coagulation.

Prenatal infections

Infections especially neonatal bacterial sepsis is the commonest cause of neonatal morality in India in which fetus may get infected in-utero and during passage through the birth canal during pregnancy and after birth. The following infections are common:

* **Intrauterine infection**	Occurs due to viruses and sometimes by bacteria causing diseases such as syphilis, tuberculosis, malaria, varicella, hepatitis B, coxsackie B, HIV, rubella, herpes simplex etc.
* **Cytomegalic**	60 to 70% patients due to this infection may suffer from bleeding, anemia, interstitial pneumonia and deafness.
* **Rubella**	About 60 to 70% patients suffer from bleeding, which may cause retardation, retinitis with pigmentation, congenital cardiac defects, valvular pulmonic stenosis, deafness and glaucoma.

* **Toxoplasmosis**	Causes severe anemia due to bleeding.
* **Congenital syphilis**	Causes rashes and snuffles, depressed nasal bridge periosteitis and chondrites.
* **Herpes virus**	Cause vesicles and pneumonia, herpes genitalia in mother.
* **Coxsackie B**	Cause respiratory distress due to carditis.
* **Congenital malaria**	Occurs due to administering infected blood.
* **Bacterial infection**	Cause blood infection, umbilical cord and ear and throat swab
* **Fungal infection (Candida)**	Causes oral and perineal moniliasis pneumonia.
* **Protozal infection**	Causes congenital malaria.
* **Spirochetal infection**	Causes rashness, snuffles, hepatitis and periostesis.
* **Viral infection**	Includes cytomegalo virus, herpes virus, vericella-zostar (chicken pox herpes zoster) influenza, measles and mumbs, which may cause vesicles, throat swab, hepatitis, anemia, deafness, cataract and cardiac malformations.

Medical interventions in labor

There are various interventions involved in labor and birth, which have benefits and risk and some of the important are described below:

- **Intravenous (IV) fluids**: The fluids are administered through plastic tube or needle inserted into the vein in the back of hand or in the arm when the patient is unable to drink liquids. Usually Pitocin is administered through IV for induce labor.

- **Prostaglandin**: A gel or tablet of prostaglandin is placed in or the cervix for 24 hours or at least overnight to soften the cervix and start labor causing uterine contractions. Most of the times this intervention fails to induce labor.

- **Artificial rupture of membranes**: Before or during the process of labor, a small hole is made in the membrane with a surgical instrument for vaginal examination before starting labor, enhancing dilation and examine color of amniotic liquid in the fetus. Sometimes, it increases the risk of infection and may increase the discomfort of uterine contractions.

- **Induction of labor**: A finger is inserted between the membranes and cervix before labor begins as light bloody vaginal discharge is often mistaken for bloody show. Labor may or may not start by this intervention. However, it may cause ruptured membranes.

- **Synthetic oxytocin (Pitocin)**: Usually it is given in an IV to cause uterine contractions to induce labor when membranes have ruptured. Oxytocin increases the intensity and frequency of contractions. In some cases it may result in incidence of jaundice in newborn or cause premature birth.

- **Fetal stethoscope**: Used to monitor fetal heart rate (FHR) and listening baby's heartbeat through abdominal wall using a stethoscope. The FHR may be counted before, during and after a contraction about 15 to 30 minutes.

- **Episiotomy**: A surgical incision made into the perineum from the vagina towards rectum just before the birth of the baby's head to enlarge the birth canal, speed the delivery of the baby, to provide more space for application of forceps or vacuum extractor and reduce compression from vaginal tissues on the head of premature baby. Episiotomy causes certain disadvantages such as discomfort in the early postpartum period, infection, frequent bleeding after delivery and pain during intercourse for several months.

- **Forceps**: A stainless steel instrument inserted into the vagina applied to each side of baby's head to aid rotation at the time of birth of head and helps to bring the baby down, reduce prolonged pressure in the birth canal and allow rapid delivery. Sometimes, the process may bruise the soft tissues of baby's head or face and vaginal tissues.
- **Vacuum extractor**: A cap like device applied to the fetal head connected to vacuum pump through a rubber tube to create suction on the baby's head. It requires less space and operational time (5 to 10 minutes) in the vagina than forceps and can be applied when the fetus is at a higher place. It may cause bruising or swelling of soft scalp tissues.

Vaginal examination when labor-pain starts

The use of abdominal palpation instead of this method of examination in normal cases has already been recommended. Where a vaginal examination is necessary it must be done with care. The patient should be on her back rather than on her side, so as to diminish the risk of the hand coming into contact with the anus. Cleanse hands and vulva before conducting the examination. The labia minora is separated apart by

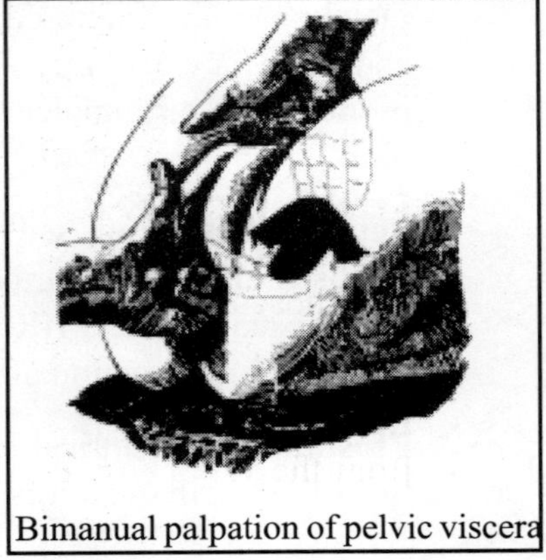

Bimanual palpation of pelvic viscera

the left hand fingers. The fingers of right hand are introduced in the vagina without coming into contact with vulva at all, or at least only the inner surfaces of the labia minora, which have also been cleansed. In case, the patient is passing through the stage of labor, it is well to introduce the fingers into the vagina during a pain and prolong the examination until it passes off. One can learn the state of matters both during and between pains. Ascertain the following points during vaginal examination:

1. State of labor; how far advanced it is?
2. Presentation and position?
3. Are the membranes ruptured? (if not, be careful not to rupture the same).
4. State of vagina and perineum to check rigidity, moistness or dryness.
5. Is pelvis normal?
6. Is cord prolapsed?

17

Important Tips for Mother & Child

Every woman needs to know the following important tips before becoming a mother

Fetus: A product of conception, irrespective of the duration of pregnancy, which is not completely expelled or extracted from its mother.

Live birth: A complete expulsion or extraction from the mother of a product of conception, irrespective of the duration of pregnancy and after such separation breathes or shows any other evidence of life such as beating of heart, pulsation of umbilical cord (movement of the voluntary muscles).

Fetal death: Death prior to the complete expulsion or extraction from its mother of a product of conception, irrespective of the duration of pregnancy. Death at a gestational age of less than 22 weeks or a fetus weighing less than 500 g o0r crown-heel length less than 25 cm is known as early fetal death. Death at a gestational age of 22 to 27 weeks or a fetus weighing 500 to 999 g or crown-heel length from 25 to 35 cm is known as Intermediate fetal death. Death at a gestational age 28 weeks or more or a fetus weighing 1000 g or more or crown-heel length of at least 35 cm is known as late fetal death. An early fetal death is called abortion, while intermediate and late fetal deaths are designated as stillbirth.

Birth weight: First weight of a live or stillborn baby taken within the first hour of life before any postnatal weight loss occurs. Babies with a birth weight of less than 2500 g irrespective of the period of gestation are known as low birth weight (LBW) babies. Babies with less than 2000 g weight are considered as high risk and are admitted to the special care neonatal unit (SCNU). Babies with a birth weight of less than 1500 g are known as very low birth weight (VLBW) babies. The babies with a birth weight of less than 1000 g are known as extremely low birth weight (ELBW) babies.

Gestational age: Age calculated from the first day of the last normal menstrual period till the date of birth (usually 34 weeks + 6 days are considered 34 weeks only).

Term: Babies with a gestational age between 37 to 41 weeks (259 to 293 days). About 10 to 12% babies are born pre-term in India. Babies with a gestational age of 42 weeks or more are classified as post-term babies. Babies with a birth weight of less than 10th percentile for their gestational age are designated as SFD babies.

Perinatal period: The period extends from the 28th week of gestation or more than 1000g to the 7th day of life. The formula for Prenatal Morality Rate (PMR) is as below:

PMR = Total prenatal deaths / Total number of births X 1000

Neonatal period: The period extends up to 28 days of life. Infant up to 28 days of life is called as a newborn baby or neonate. The first 7 days or 168 hours of life is known as early neonatal period. Period from 7 days to 28 completed days of life is known as late neonatal period.

Neonatal death: First day death occurring within 24 hours of age.

Neonatal morality rate (NMR): Neonatal death of a baby weighing over 1000 g during 28 days of life.

Maternal morality: Death of a woman known to be pregnant within 42 days of termination of pregnancy irrespective of the duration or site of the pregnancy.

Direct obstetric death: Death resulting from complication of pregnancy, childbirth or puerperium including interventions, omissions or incorrect treatment.

Indirect obstetric death: Death resulting from previous existing disease or a disease that developed during pregnancy, childbirth or the puerperium by physiological effects of pregnancy.

Incubators: These are essential to provide an ideal micro-environment of high-risk babies. The main functions of a incubator isolation are maintenance of thermo-neutral ambient temperature, desired humidity and administration of oxygen. The following newborn babies are transferred to special care nursery without delay:

- Birth weight of baby is less than 2000 g.
- Gestation of less than 36 weeks.
- Birth asphyxia.
- Rhesus iso-immunization.
- Gross congenital malformations.
- Respiratory distress.
- Maternal diabetes. Mellitus.
- Unwell or unwilling mother.

Radiant heat warmer: A portable heat lamp with two 150 Watt white ordinary or bakery bulbs or infra- red bulbs fixed on wall about 2 to 3 feet height.

Prenatal care: The health of the baby must be guarded from the day of conception. Maternal health before conception, the genetic endowments of sperms and ova, maternal infections like rubella influence the pregnancy. The ideal age of bearing children is 20 to 35 years. Take the following care:

- Smoking or chewing tobacco leaves harmful effect on the growing fetus.
- Nutritional deficiencies, if any should be corrected.

Care during pregnancy: During pregnancy the expectant mother should eat for two – for herself and for growing infant in womb. She should consume additional 25% calories as compared to her pre-pregnancy food intake and 25 g protein by taking fresh vegetables and pulses, milk and milk products. She should take regular supplements of iron and folic acid daily.

Disorders during pregnancy: These are the following:

- Pregnancy induced hypertension.
- Rhesus iso-immunization.
- Maternal infection.
- Slow growth of the fetus.
- Antepartum hemorrhage.
- Anemia (hemoglobin less than 8 g/dl).
- Abnormal presentation – unstable lie, breech presentation etc.
- Multiple pregnancies.
- Poly and obigohydramnios.
- Fetal distress.
- Cephalo-pelvic disproportion.
- Premature rupture of membranes.

- Early onset of labor.

Maternal weight: The average weight gain during pregnancy varies between 6 to 10 kg of which about 50% is contributed by weight of fetus and utero-placental unit and other half by laying-down of extra fat by the mother to provide nutritional support during lactation. The changes in abdominal girth measurement relate closely to increasing uterine size. At about 20 weeks of gestation, the abdominal girth increases by about 1 cm. every week. The average weight of placenta varies from 400-500 g (about 12-15% of body's weight).

Ultrasonography: A non-invasive, non-ionization method for antenatal diagnosis and assessment of fetal maturity, growth and malfunctions. High frequency sound waves are beamed into the woman's abdomen, placenta and all internal organs, which are transmitted onto a video screen. Gestational sac and fetal heartbeats can be identified as early as six weeks of gestation. Fetal sex can be identified as early as 8 to 10 weeks of gestation. It takes 15 to 30 minutes to get an outline of the fetus and other structures. It is safer than X-ray. An ultrasound conforms the following:

- Whether the pregnancy is uterine or ectopic.
- Estimates the age of the fetus, measures length of fetus and size of the head.
- Condition of the placenta and position of fetus in uterus.
- Confirm a multiple pregnancy.

Amniocentesis: A needle is passed through the abdominal and uterine walls into the amniotic sac and the fluid is withdrawn for examination. A local anesthesia is given to numb the skin. Amniocentesis is performed in conjunction with ultrasound. It determines the condition and placement of the fetus, placenta and umbilical cord to make a decision about continuing or terminating a pregnancy. There are several disadvantages/ risks e.g.

- Risks miscarriage.

- Injury to the fetus, placenta or cord.
- Discomfort in performing the test.
- Genetic analysis is not possible until the 14th to 16th week of pregnancy.

X-ray: Ionization radiation is used to take an internal picture of the fetus. It helps to determine the size and shape of mother's pelvis, position of the baby in womb and location of the placenta. X-ray is dangerous, since prenatal exposure to radiation has been associated with cancer and genetic mutations in babies.

Fetal movement counts: Process to record the number of fetal movements during late pregnancy. In a healthy baby the movements should be at least ten times in 12 hours. The process is simple and inexpensive but it is not fully established and a reliable procedure.

Non-stress test: Test to measure fetal heart rate (FHR) for about 30 minutes with an external electric monitor. An increase in heart rate during fetal movement is a positive sign. The test helps predict a healthy fetal and doesn't require hospitalization. Sometimes, the results are not accurate.

Contraction stress test: Also known as oxytocin challenge test. The test indicates how the fetal heart rate responds to uterine contractions. The breast nipples are stimulated until the woman has three contractions within 10 Minutes. The test is negative if the heart rate remains normal. The test is positive if FHR indicates fetal distress and in such case induced labor or cesarean delivery may be required. The test helps to determine if a risky pregnancy can be continued or should be terminated. The test is conducted in a hospital and may lead to false positive result.

Breathing after birth: Cry after the birth is not really the first breath of life because around 20 weeks of gestation, fetus starts making relatively rapid (80 to 120/min.) and ineffective respiratory movement.

How to monitor high risk factors during pregnancy? All pregnancies prone to high risk should be monitored for fetal growth, presence of congenital malformations, adequate placental functions and evidence of fetal hypoxia. The following conditions demand resuscitation alert:

- Placental insufficiency (toxemia, hypertension, diabetes, mellitus, post-maturity).
- Multi-fetal gestation.
- Poor fetal growth.
- Rhesus iso-immunization.
- Bad obstetrical history.
- Bleeding in 2nd or 3rd trimester.
- Maternal systemic disease.
- Poly obligohydramnios.
- Correct drug therapy.
- Premature labor.
- Evidence of fetal distress.
- Antepartum hemorrhage (placenta previa, abruptio placentae).
- Cord prolapse or tightness.
- Premature rupture of membranes.
- Prolonged labor (over 24 hours).
- Prolonged 2nd stage of labor (over 2 hours).
- Use of general anesthesia and narcotics.

About 15 to 20% pregnancies are complicated by passage of meconium in uterus during labor. The meconium- stained baby should never be ventilated or bagged till air passages have been effectively cleared.

Chronic systemic disorders during pregnancy:

- Bronchial asthma may be associated with fetal growth retardation.
- Chronic cardiac disease leads to premature delivery and fetal growth retardation.
- Hypertension adversely affecting the fetal growth.
- Hepatitis carries higher maternal morbidity and morality causing risk of abortion, stillbirth and pre-maturity.
- Chronic renal diseases (nephritis and nephritic syndrome) may lead to pre-mature delivery and fetal growth retardation.
- The maternal infections due to poor personal hygiene.
- Endocrinal disorders e.g. thyroid disorders, diabetes mellitus and disorders of adrenal cortex.
- Miscellaneous disorders e.g. uterine disorders, malignant disorders, epilepsy or genital factors.

Examination of baby at birth: Conduct examination undressed examination of the baby in a warm, comfortable room with baby completely undressed and placed in a flat surface having good sources of light within 24 hours of birth and check the following:

- Birth weight.
- General behavior such as color, respirations, movement of limbs and their posture.
- Skull (head circumference is more than 3 cm. bigger than chest).
- Any facial deformity.

- Skin of the body.
- Spine and other body organs.
- Feet to check any deformities.
- Abdomen and genitalia.
- Heart and chest.
- Hips to find out congenital dislocation.

Early detection of serious disease after birth: The following danger signs should be closely watched:

- Bleeding from any site.
- Appearance of jaundice within 24 hours after birth.
- Failure to pass meconium by infant within 24 hours.
- Failure to pass urine within 48 hours.
- Vomiting or diarrhea.
- Excessive crying by baby.
- Poor feeding.
- Excessive frothiness or drooling.
- Choking at feeds.
- Respiratory difficulty and/or cyanosis.
- Sudden rise or fall in the body temperature.
- Any evidence of superficial infection.

Weight record: During first year of life average daily weight gain of child is around30 g in the first month, 20 g during second and 10 g during third and fourth month of birth. Many infants double their birth weight by 4 to 5 months of age.

Immunization: The schedule of immunization is as following:

Age	Vaccine
0-7 days	BCG, OPV
6th week	OPV, DPT
10th week	OPV, DPT
14th week	OPV, DTP
9th month	Measles
15th month	MMR
18th month	OPV, DPT
24th month	TAB (2 doses at an interval of 2 weeks)
School entry	OPV, DPT, BCG
Mid school	TAB and Tetanus toxoid (every 3-5 years)

Common neonatal problems

- Vomiting.
- Failure to pass meconium and urine.
- Bowel disorders e.g. constipation and diarrhea.
- Physiological jaundice.
- Dehydration fever.
- Superficial infections.
- Excessive crying.
- Excessive sleepiness.
- Disorders due to trans-placental passage of hormones e.g. mastitis neonatrum on 3rd or 4th day, vaginal menstruation like bleeding after 3 to 5 days lasting 2 to 4 days of birth

and mucoid vaginal secretions.

- Cephalhematoma (subperiasteal collection of blood due to injury during delivery).
- Umbilical granuloma (small red flesh like nodule at the base of umbilicus with persistent discharge).
- Wetness or watering from eyes.
- Sore buttocks and napkin rashes usually due to use of nylon or tight plastic nappies.
- Various minor developmental peculiarities e.g. rashes, dry peeling skin, spots patch (stork-bites), subconjunctival hemorrhage, sucking callosities, tongue-tie, umbilical hernia and bowed legs.

Physiological handicaps

- Central nervous system.
- Respiratory system.
- Cardiovascular system.
- Gastrointestinal system.
- Thermo-regulation (hypothermia).
- Infections.
- Renal immaturity.
- Nutritional handicaps causing anemia.
- Biochemical disturbances.

Importance and advantages of breastfeeding: These include the following:

- Free from contamination and adulteration.
- Easily digestible.

- Convenient during night.
- Possesses anti-infective properties (low incidence and infective, diarrhea, respiratory infection, milk allergy and risk of eczema).
- Less likely to develop obesity and hypertension.
- Helps in spacing the birth of babies.
- Protects breast cancer.
- Promotes better figure.
- Free of cost feeding.

Biochemical and physiological difference between human and cow milk/ 100 g

Nutrients	Human milk	Cow's milk
Protein	1.1 g	3.5 g
Casein	30-40%	80%
Lactose	6.5 g	4.5 g
Fat	3.5 g	3.5 g
Ash	0.2 g	0.7 g
Cal. Phosphorus Ratio	34 mg/15 mg	122 mg/90 mg
Iron	0.29-0.45 mg	0.01-0.38 mg
Folic Acid	0.14-0.36 mg	0.01-0.06 mg
Vitamin B-12	0.0008-0.45 mg	0.07-1.15 mg
Vitamin C	1.2-10 mg	1.2-1.5 mg
Vitamin A	60-500 IU	70-220 IU

Vitamin D	0.05-10.0 IU	0.5-4.5 IU
Vitamin K	1.5 mg	6 mg

Types of breast milk

- Colostrum: Yellow thick milk secreted during the first three days after delivery, which contains more antibodies, white blood cells and contains higher protein.
- Transitional milk: Milk secreted during the following two weeks after colostrums.
- Mature milk: Milk follows transitional milk, which contains all thin watery nutrients essential for optimal growth of body.
- Pre-term milk: The mothers milk who deliver prematurely, contains more calories, higher concentration of fat, protein and sodium needed by pre-term baby.
- Fore milk: Watery and rich in proteins, sugar, vitamins and minerals milk secreted at the start of a feed, which is richer in fat content and provide more energy.

Recommendation for successful breastfeeding

- Retracted and cracked nipples must be managed before delivery.
- The first feed should be breast mi8lk. No water, honey, glucose, water, tea etc.
- Breastfeeding should be started in the first hour of life.
- Hold baby in correct position.
- Feed the baby in comfortable position.
- Rooming-in is a must for successful lactation.
- Feed baby on demand not by clock.

- Avoid bottle feed as far as possible.
- Breastfed baby does not require supplementation with water.
- Frequent suckling, emptying of breast completely, correct position while feeding and supportive care are the cause of successful lactation.

18

Breasts & Breastfeeding

In the early 1900, mostly the babies were breastfed or fed by the cow's milk. Solid foods were not offered till the age of 1 year. In 1920, people started offering solid foods. By 1975 a change had taken place, but still breast milk was more popular. Today, over 60% mothers breastfeed. Breast milk is recommended for many reasons:

- Is an ideal food for newly born babies.
- Is easily digested.
- Contains antibodies that protect the baby from infections.
- Reduces the possibility of allergic reactions.
- Aids involution and returns the uterus to its normal size.
- Makes special intimate relations between mother and baby.
- Is convenient and economical.

When breast milk is not recommended?

- If the mother has had extensive breast reduction surgery.
- The mother has hepatitis.
- Mother's breasts are infected with beta streptococcus or active herpes.
- The mother is taking drugs for cancer, seizure preventing drugs and radioactive materials.

Wearing bra during pregnancy

Ensure to make a right choice for wearing bra during pregnancy as below:

- The bra should be made of cotton and not of synthetic material.
- The bra should be well fitting o support the extra weight of the breasts during pregnancy and at the time of lactation.
- The bra should not be too tight as to compress the breasts as the pressure on breasts can harm the glands besides causing pain and irritation.
- Remove bra during night. An ideal dress a pregnant woman should wear during night is a loose gown.
- Avoid washing nipples with soap or wipe away the greasy material as this may result in soreness of the nipples. Just splash plain water to keep nipples clean.

Caring breasts during lactation

Breasts are considered an important part of a woman's sex appeal. It is important to understand what is likely to happen to the breasts for the woman breastfeeding her baby. The breasts enlarge because of the milk and the nipples enlarge and darken. The shape of breasts can be preserved if a woman take care of and wears well-fitting brassiere to support the breasts. The shape of breasts usually changes with age. Following care should be taken for breasts during lactation:

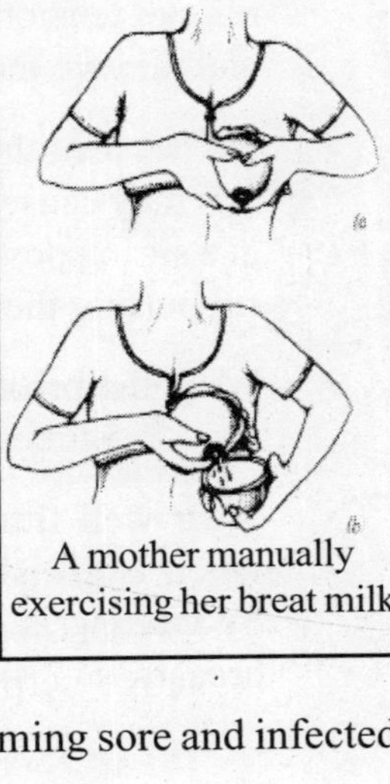

A mother manually exercising her breat milk

- Keep breasts and nipples clean and dry to prevent them from becoming sore and infected.

- Do not use soap to clean the nipples and areola; it will make them sore.
- Do not let the nipples remain moist for long; this will lead to cracking and infection.
- Keep a clean piece of cloth or a pad in your bra cup when breastfeeding to absorb leakage of milk. Make sure to change the cloth after feeding.
- Often breast nipples secrete oil. There is no need to clean the secretions from the nipples, since these protect the nipples from infection.
- If the nipples are not soft and supple, apply some cream or oil. Avoid using mustard oil as it irritates the sensitive skin. Wash the cream or oil before breastfeeding.
- Expose nipples and breasts to air daily for some time.
- Prevent engorgement of breasts by emptying them immediately after breastfeeding.
- Make sure to empty the breasts after breastfeeding to relieve tension. Press areola so that the milk comes out and remove the remaining milk with a couple of jerks.
- Do not feed the child when sleeping in incorrect posture; this may cause breast sagging. Always let the baby suckle in a sitting position with the child in the lap and your hand supporting the head.
- Wash the breasts with hot and cold baths simultaneously for 4 to 5 times daily to ensure proper blood circulation.
- Wear well fitting bra while exercising. Not wearing bra when exercising further spoil the shape of bust-line. Swimming is an ideal exercise to improve the shape of breasts.

Basics of breastfeeding

- Nurse the baby soon after the birth, this will help enhance the flow of milk and the engorgement is less of a problem.
- Get into a comfortable position. Sit comfortably supported or lie on your side. If your perineum is sore, ask for an ice bag to ease the pain and help you relaxed while breastfeeding.
- If you have had a cesarean, sitting in the bed with the baby across your lap on a pillow may be comfortable.
- Nurse your newborn in calm atmosphere, which allow you and your baby to concentrate on feeding.
- Now grasp your breast with your free hand behind the areola and compress the nipple with thumb and forefinger aligning nipple with the baby's mouth.
- Stroke your baby's cheek with your nipple. Bring your baby to your breast rather than bringing your breast to your baby.
- Let your baby suckle at e3ach breast for at least 10 minutes.
- Make sure as much of your areola as possible is in the baby's mouth to ensure a good latch.
- Arouse your baby's sense of taste by expressing a few drops of colostrums and rubbing nipples on baby's lips.
- Breastfeed on demand – every one to three hours or 10 to 15 times a day to establish an adequate milk supply.

Heavy breasts

There are no muscles in the breasts and they consist mainly of mammary glands and fat.

Mammaplasty

It is a modern cosmetic surgery, in which surgery procedure for

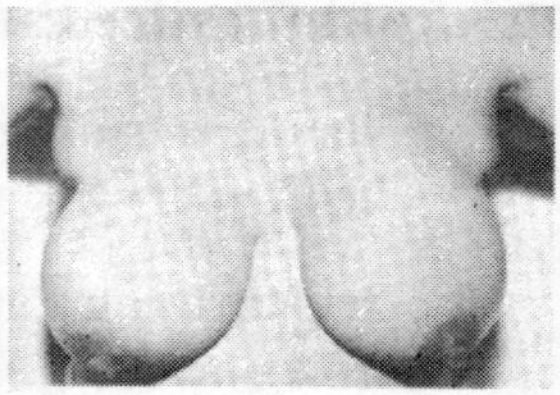

Overdeveloped Breast

breast reduction is performed to desired size in case of over-developed breasts by reducing excess breast tissue and lifting the gland if the breast sag (mastroplexy). Some people fear that breast reduction increases the chances of breast cancer. However, studies have given no evidence of it. The main cause of over-development of breasts is hyperactivity of female hormones during puberty. Sometimes, the breasts may grow to pathologically abnormal size. During pregnancy the breasts may become enlarged but regain their original shape and size after childbirth. Obese women generally have over-developed breast, which is known as 'fatty macromastia'. Women with abnormally enlarged breasts feel the following symptoms:

- Strain on cervical and thoracic vertebrae resulting in pain in the neck and backache.
- The brassiere may become a painful embodiment during menstrual period.
- Sagging breasts creates problems between the lower part of the breasts and chest wall.
- Pressure on the neck or nerve plexus due to the weight of the heavy breasts.

Breast cancer

Cancer is a malignant condition caused by abnormal rapid multiplication of cells in a part of body in women more common in cervix, uterus or breasts. According to a medical survey, out of total numbers of cancers reported over 40% are cervical cancers, 12% breast cancers, nearly 10% uterus cancers, about 10% throat cancers and rest nearly 30% The usual age to be afflicted by cancer is between 30 and 50.

Breast self-examination:

The following steps are undertaken:

- Examine the breasts standing before a mirror for symmetry in size and shape and retraction of the nipples.
- Raise arms over the head and study the breasts for similar signs.
- Recline on bed with a pillow under the shoulder on the side of breast to be examined.
- Raise arms over the head to examine the inner half of the breast. Begin at the breastbone and palpate the inner half of the breast.
- Carefully palpate the area over the nipples with flats of fingers.
- Now examine the lower half of the breasts.
- With arm down the side, examine the breast by carefully feeling the tissues extending to the armpit.
- Examine the upper outer part of the breast with the flat part of fingers.
- Finally examine the lower outer part of the breast with the flat of the fingers in successive stages.

If there is only a single nodule or lump in the breast, this is more likely to be malignant, if there is no pain. The tissue is removed by surgical procedure. In case of symptoms of cancer, immediate treatment is required. If the cancer appears to have spread to the neighboring lymph nodes, the patient should be given extensive radiation therapy to the whole affected area. Self-examination of breasts should be conducted once a month. When the cancer is present in the breast, the following symptoms are observed:

- There is usually one hard single lump with no pain.

- There may be a slight blood discharge from the nipple. Although the disease may occur at any time of life, it is much more common between the age of 35 and 60. After the age of 65, breast cancer is rare.
- Painful breasts.
- Formation of painful abscess.
- Excessive watery discharge from the nipples.

Breastfeeding problems

Difficulty with let down reflex: Anxiety, fatigue, inadequate nipple stimulation, taking excessive amount of alcohol, caffeine and smoking, especially during the hour before feeding, may inhibit the let down reflex.

Reduced milk supply: Fatigue, insufficient intake of fluids and calories or poor diet may reduce milk supply.

Poor latch: If the baby has not positioned his mouth properly on the nipple, he will be unable to compress the areola properly, and will not stimulate a let down reflex. This may lead to the baby making a clicking sound during sucking.

Engorgement: There are two causes – increased blood supply and accumulation of milk in the breasts. In such condition the following symptoms are observed:

- Swelling in the breasts.
- Breasts become hard to the touch with severe pain.

The following treatment is suggested:

- Wear a well-fitting bra during day and night for support to the breasts.
- Make sure that no area of breast is compressed.
- Apply cold pack to reduce blood flow to the breasts.

- Express milk while standing in a warm shower. Cover your breasts with warm. Moist towel.
- Express milk before feeding to soften a hard, swollen areola.
- Breast massage stimulates the milk flow.
- Use an electric or mechanical breast pump to relieve the fullness in breasts.

Flat and inverted nipples

Poor shape of nipples interferes with feeding. If the nipples appear flat or inverted, it is advised to press the areola between the thumb and the finger to help nipple to stick out and the baby will not have any difficulty in suckling. Do not apply cream or ointment on your nipples nor, it is necessary to wash them with soap.

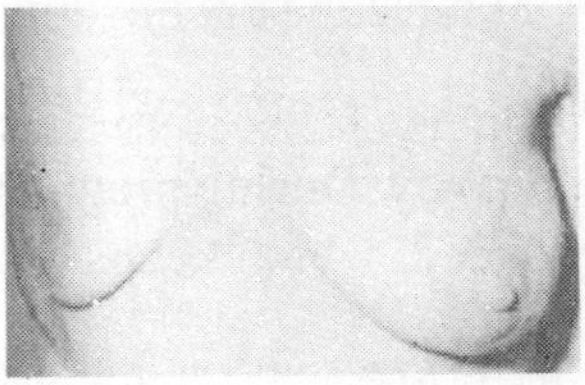

Unequal Breast

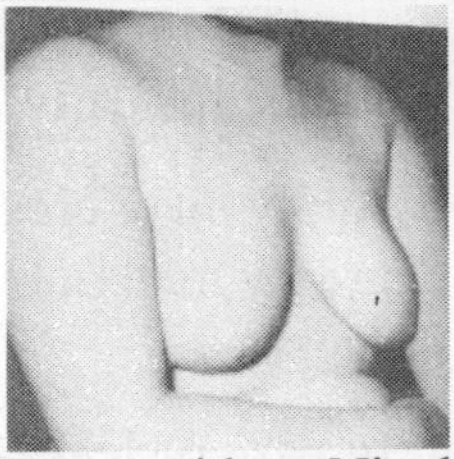

Breasts without Nipples

Cracked and sore nipples

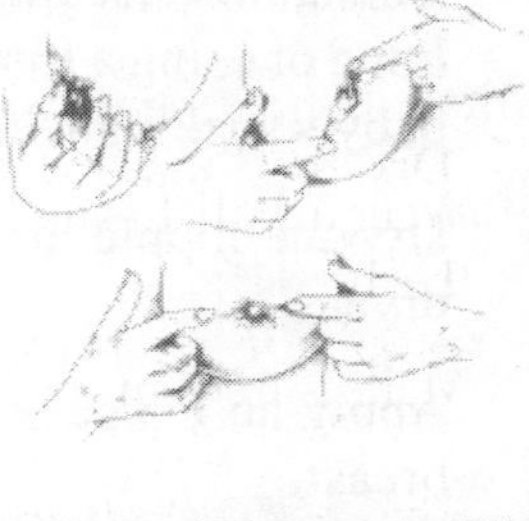

Cracks and Fixtures on Nipples

This condition occurs usually in the first week of nursing due to improper positioning of baby's mouth on the areola or poor latch. There is difference between a crack and a fissure. A fissure is generally at the base of nipple and more painful and sometimes the blood may ooze out of it. In case of a crack, a mother doesn't have to take the baby of breastfeed. To prevent crack or sore nipples the following remedies are suggested:

- Wash your breasts with plain water and keep them dry in between the feeds as wet nipples tend to become sore.
- Do not apply soap to nipples.
- Make sure that the baby's mouth is correctly positioned on your nipple.
- Feed the baby more frequently and start feeding on the less sore nipple.
- Apply oil or cream to keep nipples soft and supple. Do not apply mustard oil.
- Clean nipples after feeding.
- Expose nipples and breast to air (sunshine or sun lamp) for some time daily.
- Apply oil or cream during pregnancy. During pregnancy a greasy material is usually produced, which keeps nipples supple.
- In case of leakage of milk, use a piece of clean cloth to absorb it. Keep the cloth in cups of your bra.
- Always wear a clean bra.
- Change the feeding position very frequently. Try sitting, lying or using a foot-ball hold so that the pressure from the baby's sucking will not be in the same place all the time.
- Dry the nipple air dry with your bra flaps or set a hair dryer.
- Apply an ice pack to the sore area before feeding at the breast.
- Express a small amount of breast milk and rub it over the

sore area. Breast milk has the healing properties.

- Use a nipple shield readily available in the market in case of severe problem.

Blockage of milk in breast

The main reason for this disorder is milk of thick density unable to secrete through the blocked tube. It starts accumulating behind the blocked tube resulting in pain. Feeding mothers may also have symptoms of fever in such condition. At times, tubes get blocked because of wearing tight bras. Always wear bras, which do not exert pressure on the breasts. T is suggested that mothers suffering from this disorder should continue to breastfeed from the affected breast first so that the milk instead of accumulating and aggravating the problem drains, thus relieving the block. Massage the affected breast towards the nipple. After feeding the nipple express the breasts. You may consult a doctor if you are not getting relief. The pain and tension can be relieved by hot and cold compresses. If proper care is not taken, there are chances of mastitis suffering. In case of engorged nipple, the flow of milk in the tubes gets blocked and milk starts leaking into the infected part of the breast. In case of mastitis the infected part of the breast becomes red, painful, swollen and shiny because of stretching of the skin. However, you may continue feeding the child, because in spite of infection the germs do not pass into the milk and the baby will not suffer. A mother suffering from mastitis may develop an abscess if she discontinues breastfeeding

Epidemic Mastitis

Swelling of breasts with severe pain, a tender, reddened, hot breast, nausea, fatigue are some of the symptoms of epidemic mastitis and you should consult a doctor for the treatment and find out whether to feed the baby or not. Drainage of milk is the only remedy for getting relief from the pain. Sometimes pus may also ooze along with the milk. The patient may also have fever. The following treatment unclogs the ducts:

- Apply warm moist pack or a warm towel to the affected area.
- Massage the area towards the nipple. Perform wide circle exercise for quick relief. To do this exercise, rotate both arms five to eight times in circles without wearing a bra to strengthen the nerves and unclog ducts.
- If you have an abscess in one of the breast, you should continue feeding the baby with the other breast.
- Express milk. Make sure the mastitis breast is as empty as possible after feeding.
- Take antibiotics as prescribed by the doctor only.
- Drink lot of water, juice and other fluids
- Rest and stay in the bed as much as possible.

Expressing breast milk

There are many ways to express milk by hand or a breast pump:

- Express by hand conveniently. Once the breast is flowing, grasp your breast at the back of the areola and press towards your chest. As you compress the areola. Milk may drip or spurt into a collecting bottle.
- Breast pump is a effective equipment designed to squeeze out milk.
- Never wear anything tight or uncomfortable during pregnancy. Avoid tight bands around the waist.

19

Beautiful Body & Pregnancy

Importance of breast milk

Breast feeding a baby is one of the most valuable gifts. Breast milk is a natural, pure and unadulterated form of nourishment for the baby. It provides antibodies to the child which is why it is superior to formula feeds or cow's milk.

Why breast milk?

1. Breast feeding nurtures the emotional bonding between the mother and child.
2. It is a very convenient way to feed the baby at any place and time.
3. A breast fed baby does not require vitamin supplements as breast milk fulfils all the requirements. The nutritional quality of breast milk is much higher than that of cow's milk or buffalo's milk as it contains more lactose (milk sugar) and vitamins A,C and E. It also contains fat and iron.
4. Fat and protein in the breast milk are easily digested, thus the danger of gastro-intestinal problems is low in breast milk fed by newborn babies.
5. There is also a reduced likelihood of allergic reactions as breast milk contains protein, which does not cause allergic reaction.

Nutrition value of food you eat

A good health depends upon the nutrition value of diet we eat. To maintain good health, vigour and vitality, especially after 40 years age, a human body needs a wide range of Nutrition including Proteins, Fats, Carbohydrates, Vitamins and Minerals. These substances are derived from food we eat. The food we eat is classified as:

1. Cereals
2. Pulses
3. Legumes
4. Nuts
5. Oil seeds and grains
6. Fruits and vegetables
7. Milk and milk products

Food is grouped into two parts:

- Nutritive, which provides energy, heat and nutrition.
- Non-nutritive provides only energy, vitamins and minerals. Vitamins and minerals do not supply energy, but very important role in regulating metabolic activities. Minerals help in the formation of body structure and skeleton.

Carbohydrates:

They provide energy to the body, control break down of proteins and protect it from toxins and to burn the fat. These are found in sugar, honey, etc. Complex carbohydrates are generally found in cereals, grains, vegetables and fruits. They are more effective in controlling hunger.

Proteins:

They are various combinations of essential amino acids. They promote growth. All foods, except refined sugar, oil and fats contain proteins. Milk, oil seeds, nuts, pulses and soybean are rich source of protein, especially for growth in infants and children, fetes development during pregnancy and helps milk generation during lactation. An adult requires protein to the extent of 0.7 gm/kg of body weight. Children during growing age require slightly more proteins than adults.

Fat:

It is an essential part in human body, but it is harmful if taken in excess. Fats generally break up in the absence of carbohydrates to provide energy. Since fat is a concentrated source of energy, any excess intake of fat accumulation is termed as Obesity. The fat we eat consists of fatty acid, and is necessary for the growth and repair but accumulation of cholesterol due to fats in the body often leads to heart diseases. Eating too fat makes one obese.

1. Fasting two-three days during menstrual phase helps to provide physical, mental and psychological rest.
2. A well-balanced food with restriction on salt are essential as water rotation, before, during and after periods is quite common.
3. Drink plenty of water or warm milk to relieve fatigue and sleeplessness.

Digestive system of food

The main function of the digestive system is to break down carbohydrates, proteins and fats into simpler substances for proper absorption of the same, to keep the body systems working and also to expel the residual waste. The process of digestion is two types: mechanical and chemical. Digestion includes chewing of food, swallowing of food, churning of food, contraction of the intestinal tract and acidity reaction. There are several kinds of acid present in the food, are utilized by the body. Citric acid is present in lemons, oranges, grape fruits, tomatoes, italic acid is formed in grapes and in pineapple. Acetic acid is present in vinegar and in soy-sauce. Oxalic acid is found in spinach, rhubarb, cocoa, tea and pepper, Benzoic acid is also used as preservative, uric acid is one of the waste products of the body. Spinach, beans, peas, cauliflower and mushroom also produce uric acid. Folic acids are very useful for growth and maintenance of general health. These must be consumed by children and pregnant women as additional supplements of nutrition required by them.

Some of the important root vegetables are potato, carrot, beetroot, Jam they are rich in carbohydrates and are important source of energy, and contain vitamin C. Beans, lady's finger, tomato etc. are very low in calories and are easily digestible. Nuts and oil seeds are rich in proteins and contain high level of fat. The nutrient present in the fruits can the body obtains best. Amla and Guava contain vitamin C, Yellow coloured fruits like Mango and Papaya contain carotene. Banana and sweet lime are rich in potassium. Dried fruits such as figs, dates, raisins are rich in iron. The seeds used for extracting oils include Safflower, Sunflower, Groundnut, Coconut, gingerly and Mustard.

Vitamins and their effect

A tonic is something that invigorates, restore, stimulates or refreshes. The prominent contents of the popular tonics are vitamins and minerals. An average diet contains a sufficient amount of vitamins. The excess as well as shortage of vitamin, both are harmful and produce adverse effects:

Vitamin A: Daily requirement 3000-4000 I.U.

Available in Ghee, Butter, Egg, Fish, Green vegetables (Carrots and spinach).

Deficiency causes rough and dry skin and diminished vision. Adverse effects are headache, body aches, nausea, vomiting, itching skin and loss of hair.

Vitamin-D: Daily requirement 400 I.U. Available in fish, egg, butter, milk and sun rays. Deficiency causes decreased bone growth in children, thinning of bone in adults. Adverse effects are loss of appetite, diarrhoea, kidney failure, deposition of calcium in tissues, nervousness, trembling, headache and muscle weakness.

Vitamin B: Daily requirement 1-5 mg. Available in cereals, pulses, meat, dairy products, vegetables, nuts and fruits. Deficiency causes weakness and nervousness. Adverse effects are nervousness, trembling, headache and muscles weakness.

Vitamin B-2: Daily requirement 2 mg. Available in most foods. Deficiency causes ulcers in mouth, burning sensation in eyes and scales on skin.

Vitamin B-6: Daily requirement 2 mg. Available in meat, fish, cereals, pulses and yeast. Deficiency causes ulcer in mouth, nerve damage and anaemia. Adverse effects are pimples, skin rashes and convulsions.

Vitamin B-12: Daily requirement 2-3 mg. Available in liver, fish, egg and milk. Deficiency causes anaemia, sterility and nervous damage.

Vitamin C: Daily requirement 50 mg. Available in citrus foods, green vegetables and pulses. Deficiency causes weakness, anaemia and swelling of gums. Adverse effect are diarrhoea, kidney stone and effect on unborn baby in womb.

Nicotine: Daily requirement 20 mg. Available in liver, meat, fish, cereals and pulses. Deficiency causes diarrhoea, mental symptoms, ulcers in mouth, headache and insomnia. Adverse effects are liver damage, peptic ulcer, nausea, vomiting, diarrhoea and increase in blood sugar.

Folic acid: Daily requirement 0.1 mg. Available in liver, egg, leafy vegetables. Deficiency causes anaemia, soreness of tongue and weakness. Adverse effects are kidney damage and insomnia.

Diet during 1st and 2nd trimester of pregnancy

The first three months of pregnancy are called the First Trimester and the next three months as the Second Trimester. During the first trimester of pregnancy, a pregnant shows only a few outward signs of pregnancy, although she experiences tremendous physical and emotional changes. Throughout pregnancy, the baby in womb needs a regular supply of energy and a high quality of nutrients for its growth. It is during the first few weeks after conception that the fetes begin to form the organs and heartbeat can be detected by the second month. However, growth and maturation continues till the end of pregnancy period. The state of mind of the mother during the pregnancy affects too much over the child. Reading books, listening to music and rest makes an expectant mother happy and relaxed.

As the months roll by, the pregnant woman gets exhausted quickly. The best way to relieve tiredness and exhaustion is to ask your husband to rub your back and shoulders as a light massage on the back muscles. In case of severe nausea and vomiting, consult your doctor, who will prescribe an anti-vomiting drug. Intravenous glucose in a drip may be required if you are losing fluid every time you vomit. Have frequent small meals six to seven times in a day. Restrict your fluid intake in the evening to avoid frequent urination during the night. Eat hygienically cooked food. Relax for few minutes after meal. Avoid excess of tea, coffee and smoking.

The second trimester of pregnancy starts from the 13th week and continues up to the 28th week. The total weight gain during the pregnancy should not be more than 10 to 12 kg. During the first three months, there may be little or no increase in weight. At the end of this period there may be an increase ranging from 0.7 to 1.4 kg. or in the first 20 weeks a total of 4 kg. Make sure to watch your weight during each visit to your doctor for check up. If the weight is less than the normal gain, it indicates a poor growth of your baby in womb and you must improve your diet. If the weight is more than the normal gain, the reason could be that you are taking on excess or wrong kind of food.

Eat well balanced diet to avoid excessive weight gain. Include foods providing fibre in the diet to avoid constipation. Drink plenty of fluids and water, 7 to 8 glasses in a day. Take extra vegetables, pulses or fruits. Avoid excessive intake of sugar, salt and spices. Avoid canned and highly processed foods and avoid eating at unhygienic places. The average weight gain during pregnancy is 12 kg. Out of this, 80% is the womb and its contents. Remember, if you are overweight, there are chances of rise in your blood pressure and blood sugar.

Diet during 3rd trimester of pregnancy

During the 3rd trimester the appetite returns and mother as well as baby need a nourishing and well-balanced diet. Here is a daily diet chart recommended during this period:

Food	**Non Vegetarian**	**Vegetarian**
Milk	375-500 ml	500 ml
Meat/fish/chicken or grams/cheese		
Egg	One	
Curd	125 gm	250 gm
Whole wheat or Rice	200 gm	200 gm
Bread or cereal	50 gm	50 gm
Pulses	25-50 gm	50-75 gm
Vegetables	475-500 gm	475-500 gm
Root vegetable	50 gm	50 gm
Cooking oil/ Butter/Ghee	30-40 gm	30-40 gm
Fruits	300 gm	300 gm

Diet after delivery of child

The period after the delivery is known as postpartum and lactation. The term lactation means the secretion of milk by mammary glands (breast). During the first few days after delivery, a cloudy fluid called colostrum will be secreted in place of milk. This fluid is very beneficial for the newly born baby as it contains important antibodies to protect infant from infections and diseases. Colostrum provides adequate nutrition to the infant until the appearance of true milk after two to three days. Breast feeding is very important, it helps to build a strong bond between mother and the baby.

There is no need to panic if you do not produce a lot of milk to feed your child immediately after the delivery. It will gradually increase as you start feeding your baby more frequently. Your state of mind along with your diet influences the quantity of milk you produce. The quantity and quality of milk produced is not related to the size of breast but is dependent on the amount of diet and fluid you consume. The more often you feed your baby, the more milk will be produced. Drink plenty of juices, milk shake, buttermilk soups and water. Have minimum four litres of fluid per day while you are a feeding mother. Do not fix any rigid timing to feed your baby. Your baby will let you know when he is hungry by crying out.

Diet while breastfeeding

While breast feeding, the feeding mother will require a lot more calories than during the pregnancy. This is because breast feeding your baby will make you burn 3500 kcal per day. However you need to consume only 2400 to 2700 kcal per day during first six months of lactation if you are exclusively breast feeding your baby. Most doctors recommend that you breast feed for one year, out of this period your baby should exclusively be breastfed for 4 to 6 months, and then you can gradually start weaning by slowly introducing your baby to a variety of foods so that he is no longer fully dependent on your breast milk at the end of one year. Thus during the last six months of lactation, the energy requirement will decrease to about 2250 to 2550 kcal per day. Your diet requirement during lactation period will be as below:

- Protein: 75 gm/day during the initial six months of lactation period, which will reduce to 68 gm/day after six months.
- Fat: It is a concentrated source of energy and require 45 gm/day.
- Calcium: It is essential for the baby's development of bones as well as for the mother. The daily requirement will be 1000 mg/day. Breast milk draws calcium from the bones

in human body.

- Iron: 30 mg/day requirement is necessary to maintain haemoglobin level in the body that supplies oxygen to each cell of the body. Iron deficiency leads to anaemia.
- Folic acid: 150 mcg/day is required for the growth and development of the brain and spine of the baby. The deficiency can also lead to anaemia in the mother.
- Vitamin C: 80 mg/day is required for the formation of collagen and also for immunity against infections and diseases. Vegetables like cabbage and lettuce taken in raw form are rich source of vitamin C. Vitamin A (Beta-carotene-3800 meg/day) is required for clear vision, skin and immunity. The requirement for vitamin A increases during lactation.
- Vitamin D: It aids the absorption of calcium in body and sunlight is excellent source of vitamin D. Dietary supplements are not required.
- Vitamin B-12: The shortage is due to deficient vegetarian diets. Soya milk provides enough amount of vitamin B-12.
- During this period, your diet should include almonds, garlic, milk and fenugreek. These products increase and stimulate the production of breast milk.

How to slim without tears after delivery of baby?

A fat surplus of 10 to 15% over the normal weight must be taken as overweight. Beyond this, it is called as obesity. Over 30% it is extreme obesity. Overweight can be of three types: fatty overweight, watery overweight and cellulite.

Fatty overweight:

is really 'fat and muscle' hypertrophy, uniformly spread, accompanied by a large appetite and is common in men. The obesity is often noticeable over the upper half of the body, head, neck, arms and trunk.

Watery overweight

is a matter of 'watery fat', which does not affect the muscles at all. The obesity is most usual over the lower half of the body, and is not accompanied by any marked appetite. It is more common in women. Cellulite is a form of inflammation rather than overweight. Heredity factor, habit of overeating, ageing factor, poor functioning of system, nervous factor, sedentary life causing constipation and glandular system causing over-secretion by part of the sub-renal glands are some of the prominent causes of overweight.

To maintain a perfect figure and self grooming after becoming a mother, the amount of energy you consume must be equal to the amount of energy you burn. This includes both tangible activity and your basic metabolic rate, that is, the rate of which your body carries out its vital functions the involuntary actions of heart-beat, breathing, digestion, growth etc. which are vital to life and carry two-third of our energy intake.

- The face becomes round and bulky.
- Shoulders get plump and hollow over the collar-bones disappears.
- Fat overhang the hips and the waist disappears.
- The buttocks enlarge.
- The girdle shrinks and the rolls of flesh swell out above or below the girdle.
- The neck thickens and loses its normal contour. A double chin under the nape of the neck appears.
- Breasts sag down to the stomach.
- The stomach droops over the pubis and the pubis hangs

over the genital organs.

- The skirt belt or jean gets a little tight and there is strain on jacket buttons.

There are several causes of obesity, but the main are due to over-eating and lack of exercise. The logic way to lose weight is to cut down food intake by 100 per cent without affecting the nutritive value of the food consumed Exercise regularly to burn the extra fat. One kilogram of body fat contains 7500 calories energy. By having a daily calorie reduction of 500 calories, the total weight reduction in a month would be 2 kg.

How exercise helps?

- Tone up the muscles.
- Improve digestion.
- Increase oxygen supply to the body.
- Help to keep your weight down.
- Retain calcium in the body which delays the ageing process.
- Keep heart in good condition.
- Help glowing skin and shining hair.

The calories-controlled diets

Calories are themselves energy units and all foods contain calories to a greater or lesser amount. A normal daily diet should contain 2000 to 2200 calories to fulfil the needs of a healthy female. The protein intake should account for about 50% of your daily calories consumption. Carbohydrates should be kept to minimum. Cut down starchy foods containing sugar in favour of protein-rich foods. Lower the number of calories taken daily to about 1300 to 1600 every 24 hours.

Normally a healthy food can be digested within 15 to 20 minutes. A young woman of average height, who is not a pregnant or involved in hard physical labour, requires an average 2300 calories a day. One gram protein or carbohydrate gives four calories whereas one gram of fat gives nine calories. Protein is found in excess in milk, eggs, meat, fish, soybeans almond, coconut, groundnut etc to give strength to body. Carbohydrate is found in vegetable, fruit, cereals etc. The deficiency of carbohydrates leads to weakness. Avoid taking drastic steps in reducing weight. You are fat-prone, if you:

- Like eating.
- Have rather sedentary habits or a sedentary job.
- Put on weight during holidays.
- Are emotionally upset and worry makes you lose weight.
- Have little effect of massage and douches.

Daily requirement of calories for women doing light work is 1900. A teenager female needs daily 2200 calories. Women doing moderate work require 2200, a pregnant women 2500, a mother during lactation 2900 and a belly dancer needs 3750 calories every 24 hours. Per hour calorie consumption required by a female is given below:

- Women engaged in light household work need 120 to 300 calories.
- Women doing hard household work need 400 to 600 calories.
- Floor sweeping women require 240 to 300 calories.
- Boating consumes 125 to 220 calories in an hour.
- Swimming consumes 395 to 475 calories per hour.
- For gardening 200 to 250 calories are needed in a hour.

- Dancing consume 250 to 350 calories per hour.
- For morning walk about 150, for jogging about 800, for cycling 315 to 350 and for skating 350 to 375 calories are required in an hour.

Foods you may eat after childbirth

- Non-fatty soups and slightly salted vegetables.
- Eggs (one egg a day is sufficient).
- Fresh butter.
- Fresh or condensed milk (skimmed and unsweetened).
- Cheese with low fat contents.
- Cooked or raw green vegetables.
- Fresh fruits.
- Fruit juices and herbal teas.

Foods you should avoid after childbirth

- Bread, biscuit and pastries.
- Mutton and fatty fish.
- Fried foods, butter and oils.
- Cream and milk foods.
- Cornflakes, starchy flour and rice.
- Fatty, fermented and salted cheese.
- Banana, chestnuts, walnuts, jam, honey, cocoa and chocolates.
- Wine, beer, cider, alcoholic and sweetened drinks.

Effect of overweight on body

Overweight not only affects the looks and figure, but damages the health too, and lead to circulation troubles (Heart ailments, high blood pressure and diabetes,), psychological and nervous troubles (irritation, tiredness, nervousness, apathetic and lethargic behaviour), digestive troubles (dilation of stomach, inflammation and spasm of intestines and congestion of liver, fatty degeneration and digestive upsets) and genital disorders causing inflammation of fat into the nervous and glandular tissues which control sexual appetite, can cause temporary impotence.

Important do's and don'ts

1. Weigh yourself every 28 hours.
2. Cut down on your food intake especially bread, biscuits and cakes.
3. Use little salt and no sugar.
4. Have breakfast on one apple and tea.
5. Avoid drink while you are eating.
6. Reduce your appetite an hour before your meals.
7. Take foam bath, if possible or take a Turkish bath.
8. Exercise for 15 to 20 minutes every morning.
9. Energetic sports may keep you slim and trim.
10. Drink diuretic water.
11. Do not lose patience.
12. Do not let yourself constipated.
13. Do not take drugs without consulting a doctor.
14. Do not weigh yourself very frequently.

A balanced diet should include fruits and vegetables. These are not only rich sources of vitamins and mineral salts but are also fibre rich foods. The fibre rich diet helps our digestive system and makes heart strong. Diet should be low in saturated fats and rich in fruits, vegetables and fibres. Vegetables should form 15 to 25 per cent of daily intake, followed by fruits about 19 to 15 per cent. The dairy products and meats should not be more than 10 per cent each. Fats, oils and sweets should not be over 5 per cent in daily diet.

Have at least six to eight glasses of water every day, which flushes out toxins from the body, keeps the skin cells hydrated and helps in keeping youthful and cheerful lessening the signs of ageing. Keep strict watch on sugar and salt intake, excess of salt ends up in water retention and excess sugar is stored as reserve energy in the form of fat. Substituting sugar by 'gur' or honey is beneficial. The Calcium requirement in human body increases with the advancing age. At least two glasses of milk should be consumed daily after the age 40. Vitamin supplements should be taken under doctor's guidance as overdose of certain vitamins can lead to toxicity.

Don't neglect your body after childbirth

Daily care can help to keep your body smooth, soft and healthy. Chin, neck, upper arms, stomach, breasts, back, waistline, hips, thighs and bottom are some of the areas of the body which require special care by every woman to maintain her personality and improve skin texture, colour and tone.

Beauty of Neck:

Neck is the most neglected area of body. Whenever, having facial, include neck in all facial routines such as cleansing, toning, moisturizing and nourishing. Use a special nourishing cream during night before sleep and gently massage. Massage and exercises reduce extra fat on neck. In winter, massage with nourishing or cold cream mixed with a little almond oil.

Beauty of Waistline:

A slim waistline makes a woman highly appealing. Waistline lends flexibility to her frame and enhance gait. Generally hip-bone of a woman is much broader than the man, especially after the delivery of child. One develops fattening tendency and the waist becomes flabby losing its natural beauty. Here are few suggestions for the attraction of waistline:

1. Massage with olive oil to prevent wrinkles, flabbiness and folds during pregnancy and after delivery on waistline.
2. Walk, rope jumping, dance and swimming are important exercises for the waistline.
3. Avoid use of high pillow, it deforms and weakens waist.
4. Use hard bed without foam mattresses.
5. Do not rely on false advertisements claiming to restore your slim waistline by the use of belts or corsets.

Hips and thighs

Apart from having a beautiful face, if your body is disproportionate, you will lose all its charm. To have a check on your posture, arrange a mirror in such a way that you can see your side view completely. If your arms fall along the back line of your hips, then you stand with your stomach protruding. Correct your posture by holding your stomach in, so that the arms fall in the centre of the side of the body. Now if your arms fall in front, then you have probably protruding hips. Therefore, try to reduce weight on the hips, and also bring the waist and the back a little backwards. Make effort to push the hips forward, till your arms fall in the centre of the side of your body The body should meet the following measurements:

Bust	6 times your wrist
Waist	4 times your wrist

Hips	6-1/4 times your wrist
Thighs	3-1/2 times your wrist
Calves	2-1/4 times your wrist
Ankles	1-1/2 times your wrist

Hips and thighs are adversely affected after deliver of baby. Fat hips and flabby thighs spoil the gait. It is important to be alert immediately after the delivery, otherwise it will be too late. It is a gradual process and hence beauty-conscious women recognise the signals at the very beginning and take steps to keep body proportionate.

Every woman must know the required proportions of her thighs and hips according to her height as given below:

Height (cm)	**Hips (cm)**	**Thighs (cm)**
153	85	47
155	86	49
158	87.5	51
160.5	89	52
163	91.5	53
165.5	94	56

Sagging buttocks

The sign of sagging affects buttocks which start sagging due to Lack of muscle tone, lack of support and elasticity in the skin. Regular massage with anti-cellulite oils can help break down the fatty deposits underneath the skin. There are several reducing creams available in the market to massage the buttocks but they do not work deep down enough to work up or decrease the size of buttocks.

However, exercises specifically for the buttocks will help.

Stomach

Stretch marks on stomach are caused due to fibre beneath the skin surface weaken and the normal elasticity of the skin is not enough to bear the weight or excess fat. These marks mostly occur after the childbirth and sometimes appear in puberty when the growth rate of the body is fast. Apply olive or baby oil throughout pregnancy and immediately after childbirth. Lubricating the skin as a part of daily routine helps to minimise these stretch marks. The marks may also fade a little with regular application of a cream containing a large concentration of vitamin E. More serious stretch marks require surgery. Exercises stimulating stomach muscles will help.

Breast beauty

If you have mottled-looking skin on the breasts, stimulate circulation with alternative rinse of hot and cold water, it will help to minimise the problem and make your bosom firmer. If the skin looks wrinkled and sagging particularly when you are feeding a baby, use a good moisturising cream. Breasts require maximum attention after delivery. Breasts usually sag, if the infant is suckled while sitting in a faulty posture. Suckling with the infant in lap or suckling lying down both are harmful for breasts. Do not forget to press nipples immediately after breastfeeding and remove the remaining milk with a couple of jerks, this gives lightness and freshness to the breasts.

Back

Spotty back are often a problem for people who tend to have greasy or combination facial skin. The over-active sebaceous glands that cause the secretions which start the spots are themselves stimulated by hormonal activity in the body, particularly in adolescence. The only remedy is to keep the skin scrupulously clean by washing with a medicated liquid soap daily and by changing the clothes. To avoid unnecessary irritation, choose cotton for the vest, bra, blouse or T-shirt. Apply medicated cleansing lotion and anti-acne cream to dry up the excess grease at bed-time. If a spot appears on the back, just before you plan to wear a low-backed or backless dress, disguise it with a medicated make-up matching your skin tone. Here are few tips for the back:

1. As far as possible use medicated soap to heal rashes.
2. Massage back with mustard oil before taking bath.
3. Rub anti-acne lotion at night.
4. Wear loose dresses to avoid itching.
5. Rubbing lemon on the skin of back clears the skin of its dark patches usually appears during pregnancy. Rubbing lemon is also effective for a dark complexioned skin. Cut a lemon in two pieces, rub on the back, let juice dry for ten minutes followed by washing off with cold water.
6. If you have unwanted hair on the back, this can be hidden by bleaching. Use a face pack on the back, which ensures a beautiful, soft, lustrous skin. Mix to it few drops of hydrogen peroxide and mustard oil in the pack.

Bottom

Bottoms are sun and air starved, and even in summer these are covered, so tend to look pale and pasty. Nude sun-bathing is impractical for Indian women but instead of that you can use ultraviolet lamp for few seconds everyday. Bottom is also adversely affected during pregnancy and during labour-pains. Use plenty of body lotion and moisturiser on this area. Pinching the flesh on bottom when you are in bathing tub is good for circulation and shape and reduces extra flesh.

Honey massage for cracked nipples of breasts

Mix one teaspoon each of honey and olive oil (or lanolin). This is very useful to apply on cracked nipples. This oil massage soothes and softens the skin of breasts.

Ten steps to get rid of flab after childbirth

Mind set: The success of your weight reduction fairly depends on your will power, keenness and attitude - without which nothing really works.

Right aim: Looking to lose immediately is an unrealistic and unreasonable goal. Aim to reduce weight gradually, not quickly.

Exercising: Make exercise an integral part of your daily routine. Brisk walking, cycling, playing tennis or badminton, swimming, aerobics and yoga exercising are some of the easy exercises, Start up with a 10-minute routine and gradually increase it to 30-40 minutes daily.

Change in lifestyle: Lifestyle changes are must. If you are having sedentary habits, you are likely to lose more than gain. Avoid making obesity, a way of life. Walk briskly, take to the stairs instead of riding the lift or a elevator are good habits.

Diet control: Exercise control over your diet to lose weight. Remember, crash dieting is unhealthy, though it works well initially but leaves worse effects. You put on whatever weight you had lost. Eat slowly, avoid going to a party on an empty stomach, Eating an low or no-fat diet and consuming more of fibre-rich and unrefined foods are some of the good habits.

Don't skip meals: Skipping a meal and ending up eating more at the next meal is rather harmful.

Avoid late dinner: Watch what you eat after 7 pm, as the food you eat late is stored in the body as pure lard. Food enters the blood stream as energy after four hours of taking dinner. Since the body does not need energy, so the food is stored in the fat cells as fat. As far as possible, have light dinner.

Release toxins: Water helps washing away the toxins from the body. Start the day with a glass of water.

Skip meal: If you feel hungry in the evening, snack up but skip dinner. If you had a heavy lunch, then just take a bowl of soup for dinner.

Maintain food diary: In spite of diet control, if you have not reduced at all although visiting a gym or a health club regularly, then maintain a food diary. Make a record of everything you eat or drink from you wake up early morning till night you go to bed for two weeks. You will find your wrongs.

Obesity

Obesity is not a disease in itself but it is at the roots of many diseases like high blood pressure, heart trouble, diabetes, kidney trouble, gout, joint pains, stone and skin diseases. As stated earlier, many causes of obesity include overeating, lack of exercise and lethargy, heredity, overactive lands in the body (which increase appetite), an imbalance of hormones in the body, mental tension, frustration, loneliness and after-effect of childbirth.

Physical adjustments during postpartum

After baby's birth, mother feel exhausted, fatigued and let down and her body undergoes rapid physical and hormonal changes. For early recovery very frequently check your temperature, pulse, respiratory rate, blood pressure and monitor the amount and character of lochia (red-coloured, fleshy-odour discharge from vagina flowing heavily for the first day after the birth of baby, which diminishes in a week's time changing its colour to pale pink in next 3 to 4 days and finally becomes yellowish white or brown with the presence of bloody clots for 6 to 8 weeks). Avoid infection or over-exertion, which cause excessive bleeding. In such case consult your doctor. There are few more problems faced by the mother during postpartum period as below:

After-pains: Painful contractions of the uterus occur. To cope with the pain relax and use the slow-breathing pattern. After-pains may disappear after a week.

Cervix conditioning: The cervix shrinks to its pre-pregnant size but remains somewhat wider for few months.

Vaginal toning: The vagina gradually regains its tone, but the labia remain looser, larger and darker as compared to pre-pregnancy condition.

Breasts: Breasts secrete colostrums (a yellow fluid that precedes breast milk). The milk production starts between the 2nd and 5th day after the delivery. During this period the breasts may feel tense, hard to the touch and painful (engorged). Non-breastfeeding mothers still produce milk. To suppress lactation, breast binding, ice packs and avoidance of breast stimulation help diminish milk production. Do not express milk from breasts, this will stimulate the breasts to produce more milk.

Circulatory changes: Some blood loss is natural after childbirth. Average blood loss amounts to approximate one cup in normal delivery, but may be double in case of an episiotomy. Slight blood lost during the childbirth is not harmful, but if blood losses are more consult a doctor.

Stretch marks and pigmentation of abdominal skin: After the birth, the abdominal muscles remain soft for about six weeks and stretch marks appear. These marks fade with the passage of time but do not disappear completely. However, skin pigmentation will fade away after few months.

Hormonal changes: After childbirth the body undergoes sudden and dramatic changes in hormonal production. The hormonal producing level drop abruptly and remain low until ovaries begin producing these hormones again. If a woman breast feed, she may not menstruate for several months, though ovulation can occur during this time. However, if a mother is not breastfeeding, she will begin menstruating within 4 to 6 weeks after the birth. First few menstrual periods following delivery may be heavier than usual, but will return to normal soon.

Rest and activities: Adequate rest is essential to recover after childbirth. Try to rest an extra two hours daily and go to bed early at night.

Exercise: Perform the pelvic floor contraction exercise (known as Kegel) to heal episiotomy or any tear, reduce the swelling and restore the muscle tone in the pelvic floor. Try to begin postpartum exercises within a day or two in case of a normal delivery. Better consult your doctor in this regard. The conditioning exercises during pregnancy help you recover former contours and strength during the postpartum period. Two areas of the body: abdominal muscles and pelvic floor muscles (to reduce swelling, increase circulation and promote healing in the perineum and restore vaginal muscle tone) need special attention Here are few postpartum exercise:

- Gently tighten and then relax the muscles of perineum several times a day for pelvic floor contraction.
- Lie flat in bed with knees bent. Tighten abdominal muscles to tilt the pelvis pressing low back into the bed. Pelvic tilts can be performed while standing or sitting also.

Uterus examination: Fundus can be felt midway between the navel and the pubic bone. Massage the uterus, which helps to maintain the firmness of uterus, prevent heavy blood loss from the placental site and return to its previous size. By the end of 5 to 6 weeks, the uterus returns to its previous size.

Sexual adjustments: Some men and women want to resume sexual intercourse as soon as possible after the birth, though most of females feel constrained or afraid and lack enjoying making love due to a sore perineum and extreme fatigue. If you are not ready to resume intercourse early, you may resume pleasuring (touching and enjoying each other's bodies sensually with or without orgasm). It is suggested to refrain from intercourse for at least six weeks after the birth. It is, however, safe to have intercourse when stitches heal, vaginal discharge stops and you feel like it. There is decrease in vaginal lubrication after childbirth because of hormonal changes. The problem can be alleviated by use of a sterile, water soluble lubricant such as K-Y jelly or contraceptive cream during intercourse. Remember, conception can occur whether or not menstruation has resumed. The condom along with spermicidal foam, cream or jelly is safe and effective method after childbirth.

20

All About Menstruation Menopause & Anemia

Menstruation is a periodic change occurring in human consisting of discharge of blood from the cavity of the womb. It usually starts between 12 to 13 years in warm climates and later in cold regions with duration of each menstrual period varying from 2 to 8 days. There is an interval of 21 to 28 days between the two periods. The menstrual flow stops when a woman becomes pregnant. It stops completely at the age of about 50, when it is known as the menopause. The two main disorders of menstruation:

- Absence of periods or scanty and painful discharge known as amenorrhoea and dismenorrhoea.
- Profuse bleeding during periods known as menorrhagia or irregular menstruation called as metrorrhagia.

Amenorrhoe

Scanty discharge of menstrual blood or absence of menses flow may be due to

- Anemia.
- Ill health.
- Disturbed nervous system.
- Imperfect development or functioning of ovaries.
- Inflammation of various internal organs (womb, ovaries or

fallopian tubes).

- Serious or prolonged diseases like tuberculosis, aggravated dyspepsia malaria etc.
- Sudden fright or great grief, which may cause stoppage of the menstrual flow for months. Steep 1 tablespoon each sesame seeds and small Caltrops (gokhru) in 200 ml water. Sweeten with sugar or honey and drink.
- Do not over-strain yourself mentally or physically.
- Hot and cold hip bath and sunbathing will be beneficial.
- Fasting for 2 to 3 days during menstruation is advisable to provide physical, mental and psychological rest.
- A well- balanced food with restriction on salt is essential as water retention before, during and after menstruation is quite common.
- Drink plenty of coconut water, barley water, 'dhania' water or butter milk, which have diuretic effect. Drink a glass of warm water with honey before going to bed , which relieves fatigue and induces sleep.

Dismenorrhoea

The symptoms in this case include:

- Pain during menstruation flow.
- Vomiting sensation during periods.
- Feeling of weakness generally due to inflammation of internal organs e.g. the womb, ovary defects or malfunctioning and fallopian tube. The following herbal remedies are helpful to treat this menstruation disorder:
    1. The leaves of the herbs Indian wild pepper (sambhalu), horse radish, (sahinjana), Indian lilac (bakayan), wild chicory (kasni), black night-shade (mako), marsh-

mallow (khatmi), cotton plant (narma kapas) and dill (soya) are boiled in water.

2. The leaves are cooked in sesame oil, dried and tied on the lower abdomen like a poultice.

Menorrhagia

It is the excessive discharge of blood from the womb during periods usually due to faulty functioning of ovaries. The following remedies help:

- Amla should be soaked in juice of green amla for three days and then ground into powder. Take this powder with milk.
- An hot and cold hip bath is very beneficial for menorrhagia patients.

Some facts about heavy bleeding during menstruation

- Heavy bleeding during the childbearing age may be due to miscarriage or abortion or as a result of an ectopic pregnancy. Tumor of uterus and cervix may result in vaginal bleeding. Women with irregular or very heavy bleeding should consult a doctor and have a Pap test every six months.
- A careful examination for the presence of cancer should be conducted by scrapping the inner lining of the uterus. Intermittent spotting may be due to cervical polyp – a common condition in women over 40. Heavy bleeding may be due to fibroid tumors and polyp within the uterus. In some cases either the tumor or perhaps the entire uterus may have to be removed.
- If a woman is in mid-pregnancy and starts bleeding, she should be rushed to the doctor. It may be too late to save the child in the womb. Severe blood loss may cause a danger to the life of woman.

- Heavy or painful bleeding is common in younger women due to various conditions such as blood diseases, alcoholism, cirrhosis of the liver, vitamin B deficiency and abnormalities either in thyroid, pituitary or adrenal glands causing heavy bleeding. A complete medical examination including a careful evaluation of pelvic organs have to undergo. In such case a complete bed rest, a high protein diet and multi-vitamin capsules are recommended. If the woman has lost excess quantity of blood, a transfusion may be needed. Heavy bleeding following abortion usually requires a surgical operation to clean out from the uterus any fragments of the placenta still present in the uterus.
- During teenage, girls become depressed at the though of painful periods, which is not abnormal and such girls should indulge in normal activities and there is no reason for them to go to bed for two to three days every month due to this indisposition
- During teenage years young people suddenly become conscious of sex and striking changes take place within the body. Bad company and lack of p-roper guidance may lead to a life of sorrow and tragedy. A female should understand that her monthly cycle has a beneficial effect on her body. Menses may be irregular at first, but this is nothing to worry about. Some teenage girls have periods as early as 11 years of age, others do nor begin until their 16 year, yet all are perfectly normal.

Leucorrhoea

Leucorrhoea or whites is a symptom of many diseases peculiar to women. It consists of white watery discharge from the uterus, which may be thick consisting mainly of pus if the patient is suffering from a serious disorder of the genital organs. Leucorrhoea discharge may be of several types as below:

- In most cases the discharge is catarrhal and chronic in

nature.

- In few cases the discharge follows or precedes the menstrual flow.
- In sever cases the discharge continues throughout the intervening period.
- The patients suffering from leucorrhoea have the following symptoms:
- Look pale and unhealthy.
- Feel tired at slight exertion.
- Have constant pain in lower back.
- During early adolescence and teen years, increased white discharge combined with itching is common due to infection immediately before and after the periods.
- During the mid-cycle, white discharge increases when ovulation occurs.
- The discharge increases during pregnancy.
- During sexual excitement, there is excessive vaginal wetness.
- In anemia and other general rundown states of health, the white discharge increases.
- Vaginal discharge and irritation increases because of bacterial or fungal infection due to vaginitis.
- There is always excessive vaginal discharge in ease-loving women, neither do household work or exercise their body. Manual workers are less susceptible to leucorrhoea.

Remedies:

- Avoid wearing tight synthetic undergarments..
- Avoid use of strong antiseptics.

- Clean the genital parts once or twice a day to prevent vaginal infection.
- In case of husband has urinary infection or suffering from trichomonasis or candidiasis, he will have to be treated along with the wife, otherwise she would get re-infected repeatedly.
- Avoid highly spiced foods.
- Exercise the body by running, playing or getting involved in household work.
- Have sunbath daily for 15 to 20 minutes.
- Cold compress applied to the vagina helps a lot. A cold compress may be worn like a sanitary towel for an hour or may be worn during sleep.
- In young girls the discharge may be due to irritation of the labia or external genital organs, over-activity of sex glands and organs, due to soiled under garments, dirt and intestinal worms and masturbation.
- In mature women, sometimes profuse yellowish discharge associated with urination may be due to venereal diseases (usually gonorrhea) or presence of creamy, slightly blood-stained discharge due to cancer in the uterus or cervix.

MENOPAUSE

A female becomes reproductive in early teens and can bear a child till her mid or late-forties. After passing through various stages of her sex life, a woman enters menopause, which marks the end of her fertile period and beginning of a new phase. When periods finally stop and fertility ceases, menopause sets in. At the beginning of menopause, the usual complaints include the following:

- Hot flushes.
- Dizziness and fainting.

- Lack of energy and depression.
- Fainting, burning feet and hands.
- Vaginal dryness.
- Loss of sleep.
- Severe itching.
- Facial hair growth.
- Sudden increase in weight.
- Mental tension.
- High blood pressure.
- Complete loss of interest in sex.
- Palpitations, chilly feeling and constant backache arising from low levels of estrogen in the blood stream.
- Imbalanced hormonal levels.

Gout and leg cramps during menopause

Gout is a type of arthritis causing throbbing pain that often strikes quite often at night in pregnant women during the last trimester of pregnancy as well as during menopause. The skin turns red and hot, leaving the affected joint swollen and tender. Gout is caused by uric acid crystals, which settle in joints. Often the big toe is the prime target of its effect. Doctors usually inject very toxic drug to stop pain by dissolving uric acid crystals or prescribe ibuprofen (800-milligram) for relieving pain. The following curative measures are suggested to treat gout:

- If the affected joint is not too tender, try applying a crushed ice pack placing on the painful joint for about ten minutes.
- Avoid taking high-purine foods (include high protein animal products and sweet bread, dry beans, whole-grain cereals and yeast) that contribute to higher levels of uric acid.

- Drink lot of water to flush out excess uric acid from body system.
- Avoid taking alcohol if you have a history of gout. Alcohol increases uric acid production in the body, which get deposited on joints.
- Eating cherries prevents production of uric acid.
- Vitamin B 6 helps distribute water in the body to keep its all tissues hydrated, which helps prevent uric acid from turning into crystals.
- Taking a tablespoon of apple cider vinegar in the morning daily is very effective to prevent gout attacks.
- Mix charcoal into a bath and soak affected foot in it for 30 to 60 minutes. Mix ½ cup of charcoal powder in water.
- Persons with high blood pressure should control the blood pressure when they suffer from gout.

Leg cramps in the calves or feet commonly occur in women, especially in late pregnancy when she is resting or asleep. Cramps are usually caused by the factors, such as fatigue in calf muscles, pressure on the nerves to the legs, impaired circulation and calcium-phosphorus imbalance in the blood. Cramps are relieved by the following measures:

- The muscle is slowly and gently stretched.
- Gently stretch calf muscles. Keeps knees straight, ankles bent and heels resting on the floor. When the leg cramp is severe you may need help.
- A foot cramp, which usually tightens the muscles of the arch and curls the toes can be relieved by stretching out toes. To prevent cramping do not curl your toes.

What is Menopause?

Menopause-usually around the age of 50 is called 'The Change' when functioning of ovaries to produce eggs, the swelling and bursting of the egg sac, release of the hormones (estrogen secretion), monthly menstrual shedding of uterine cells and blood becomes irregular and slowly comes to a halt. The prominent symptoms during menopause include hot flashes and sudden chills, lowered sexual desire, emotionally upset, insomnia, depression, memory loss and sudden change in the mood and night sweating. Sometimes, the sweating is so high you may have to change the bed sheet.

The following measures make better outlook of life during menopause:

- Make life an adventure. Find a new hobby and change in the career.
- Daily exercise should be a part of your daily life. Walking, jogging, bicycling, jumping rope, dancing, swimming or any other daily exercise can relieve menopausal disorders. Yoga aids relaxation and reduces stress.
- Hot flashes are body's response to lower estrogen levels and more than 75% women usually have hot flashes lasting between two to three minutes. During excretion of hot flashes, heat is produced in the body, the face reddens and there is excessive sweating.
- Nutrients can help control or completely eliminate hot flashes. Vitamin A is as effective as estrogen (recommended daily dose 400 to 1200 international units as recommended by your doctor). In case of night sweats, have two doses during the night as per suggestions of your doctor.
- Vitamin E helps in case of vaginal dryness.
- Learn meditation or yoga or sit quietly, eyes closed to relax

your mind.

- Alcohol triggers hot flashes. Similarly cut down caffeine containing beverages that stimulate production of the stress hormones and trigger hot flashes.
- Wear fiber clothes. Synthetic fiber trap heat and produce perspiration during a hot flash.
- Drink lot of water or juice, especially after exercising to check body temperature.
- Eat small meals-minimum three meals a day. Even five to six small meals a day will help your body regulate temperature more easily.
- Vitamin B complex helps to reduce stress in menopausal women.
- The herb sage works very well if menopausal woman have hot flashes throughout the day and sweat during night. Drink a sage tea.
- Hydrotherapy treatment is very helpful for menopausal women. The body expels toxins during menstruation. When menstrual cycle decreases or stops the body requires another outlet for the toxins, so it starts sweating or has hot flashes. It is advised to have sauna (steam) bath to release toxins from the body. In case a sauna or steam room is not possible, take a hot bath for 10-20 minutes a day.
- Valerian and lavender herbs help better sleep. Take 300 to 500 milligrams valerian extract one hour before retiring to bed at night. Dabbing a few drops of lavender essential oil on your pillow before sleep can help you a sound sleep.
- Acupressure therapy relieves insomnia and anxiety in menopausal women. Stimulate two pressure points on the feet for 1 to 3 minutes each with your middle and index fingers.

- Women passing through their menopausal period if stay sexy and have regular intercourse once a week or once a fortnight have few or no hot flashes or night sweating as compared to those women who doesn't indulge in sexual intercourse at all. Having frequent sex helps moderate drop in estrogen levels, which reduce hot flashes. A study reveals that regular sexual activity stimulates the functioning of ovaries.
- Vaginal dryness from a lack of estrogen decreases interest in sexual intercourse among menopausal women. Lubricants suitable for vaginal dryness include vaginal jelly, vegetable oil and unscented cream or oil.
- Vitamin E can be used to massage as a lubricant. Break open vitamin E capsules and mix to the lubricant

Anemia

Anemia-an iron deficiency in the body is a problem that affects every one out of five women. Anemia is a condition in which the blood has too few red cells, which results in a lessened ability of the blood to supply oxygen to the tissues resulting in weakness, lassitude and pallor. Iron-deficiency anemia may cause symptoms,

Such as dizziness, loss of appetite, diarrhea, abdominal pain, pale complexion, palpitation of the heart, shortness of breathe, feeling of weakness and frequent headache. The blood needs iron to produce red blood cells. Women who don't get enough iron in their diets or who have heavy menstrual periods may have insufficient levels of either red blood cells or hemoglobin, the oxygen carrying protein in red blood cells. Women whose hemoglobin level decline feel tired and weak. If you have excessively heavy or lengthy menstrual flow or your menstrual period lasts for more than seven days, you should consult a doctor. If you are having rectal bleeding, you need to see a doctor. Improve your diet and lifestyle in order to have a healthy baby and trouble-free delivery of child.

How to find that you are anemic?

Press your unpolished fingernail against the nail bed for few seconds. The area will turn white. Then stop pressing, if the nail area turns pink very slowly and takes time, you have anemia. By having a complete blood count performed by a competent laboratory, it can be observed that a man or a woman is anemic. Skin color cannot confirm that he or she is anemic. Many people who seem, to be pale have normal red blood cells and are not anemic at all. However, it is common for females in the age group that menstruate. The loss of blood during periods must be replaced by new blood produced in the bone marrow. This required that the woman have enough iron in her diet. In case of un-sufficient iron contents in diet she may become anemic.

What is blood?

Blood is the fluid circulating through blood vessels. It contains red blood cells, platelets and a pale yellowish liquid known as plasma. Plasma acts as a fluid medium for the suspension of blood cells., transports dissolved nutrients to the tissues, carries waste products from tissues to the organs. The red blood cells contain hemoglobin and red pigment of the blood. The oxygen is thus carried to all the tissues of the body. The white blood cells known as leukocytes, which act as body's defense again infection and combat fighting against bacteria and viruses. They also produce proteins called antibodies, which fights infection. Platelets are circulating cells that prevent and stop bleeding

Few remedies for anemic women

- Have iron-rich food. Good sources of iron include whole grains such as barley and oats, beans and peas, seeds and nuts, fruits and vegetables.
- Calcium rich foods put more iron in your body. Dairy products decrease iron absorption in women with anemia,

whereas increase your intake of beans, peas, soybeans, sesame seeds, soups and leafy green vegetables. Inadequate diet is one of the most common causes of anemia.

- Vitamin C is acidic and helps the body to absorb iron contents. Squeeze the juice of a lemon into a glass of water and drink before meals. Alternatively, take vitamin C (1,000 to 2,000 milligrams a day with each meal).
- Remember, alcoholic beverages (wine and beer) deplete the body of vitamin B complex and minerals, which can worsen anemia. Reduce your sugar intake, which also depletes the body of vitamin B complex.
- Delete caffeine (products such as coffee, black tea, soda, chocolate etc.) from your daily diet, which depletes the body of vitamin B complex.
- If the anemia results from iron deficiency, iron pills are suggested. But if the anemia is associated with vitamin B-12 deficiency, the vitamin must be administered by injection.

Types of anemia

Sickle-cell anemia: Usually characterized by a chemical abnormality of the hemoglobin, which results in the sickle-cell shape of the cells. The cells do not survive and circulate and the patient becomes anemic. In this case a severe anemia is present and children (including older children) with this condition are usually jaundiced, may have long, thin arms and legs and a protruding abdomens as a result of blood not circulating thoroughly in the body. To treat sickle-cell anemia, blood transfusions are given to restore red cells. Doctors recommend antibiotics to protect against infection. Good nutrition, plenty of fluids and vitamins help to improve condition. A female or a male suffering from sickle-cell anemia may get marry but they need genetic counseling before having a child.

Deficiency anemia: Usually caused by lack of a substance necessary for the formation of blood.

Pernicious anemia: It results from vitamin B-12 deficiency. Such women should take vitamin B-12 throughout the life.

Iron-deficiency anemia: It is caused by acute or chronic loss of blood. Such anemia can be treated by blood replacement by giving iron pills, which produce red blood cells.

Congenital anemia: This type of anemia occurs in women born with defective blood in the body. Blood cells usually are destroyed in the body.